Universal Yoga®

4 x 4 Universal Yoga® Mandala Sequence

(Second Edition)

Written by

Suresh Munisamy

and

Andrey Lappa

Edited by

Sheri Baemmert

TABLE OF CONTENTS

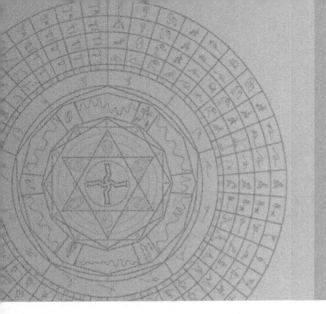

FOREWORD

Suresh Munisamy has spent many years practicing yoga in India, and he has already been teaching Universal Yoga® for over five years.

Being born and growing up in India he knows very well the real meaning of Yoga as an authentic spiritual path. That is why he found Universal Yoga® as a form of authentic Yoga for himself and became one of the leading Universal Yoga® teachers in Thailand.

The moral qualities of the practitioner are very important in traditional Yoga. Suresh always presented himself as a respectful, well-educated, hard-working and advanced practitioner when he was studying with me and during our informal communication. I highly love and respect Suresh personally, and he is very dear to me as one of my best students and Universal Yoga® teachers in the world.

I was impressed by the good quality and fast work which Suresh did writing this book, and I hope it is just a beginning for Suresh's even greater publications in Universal Yoga® in the future. I know that Suresh's first yoga book will benefit many Universal Yoga® practitioners in the world for the years ahead.

The Yoga path of self-perfection has no limits. And with all the perfect qualities of the Universal Yoga® practitioner and teacher which Suresh has already, I hope he will never stop practicing, teaching, and reaching the highest levels of personal results and enlightenment.

I know that Suresh is representing Universal Yoga® and Shiva Nata® authentically and with perfect form. And I recommend that all students interested in Universal Yoga® and Shiva Nata® study with him in any countries where he teaches.

Andrey Lappa

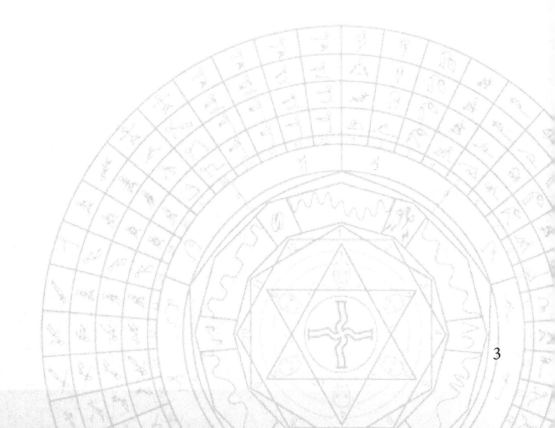

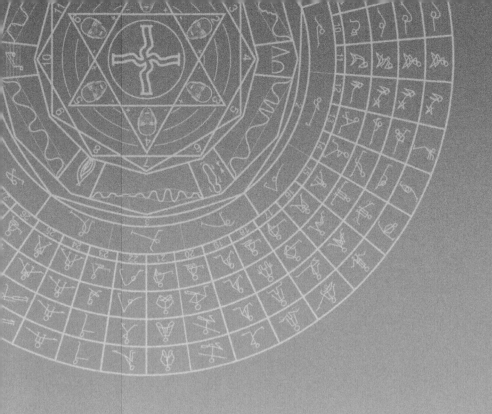

INTRODUCTION TO YOGA

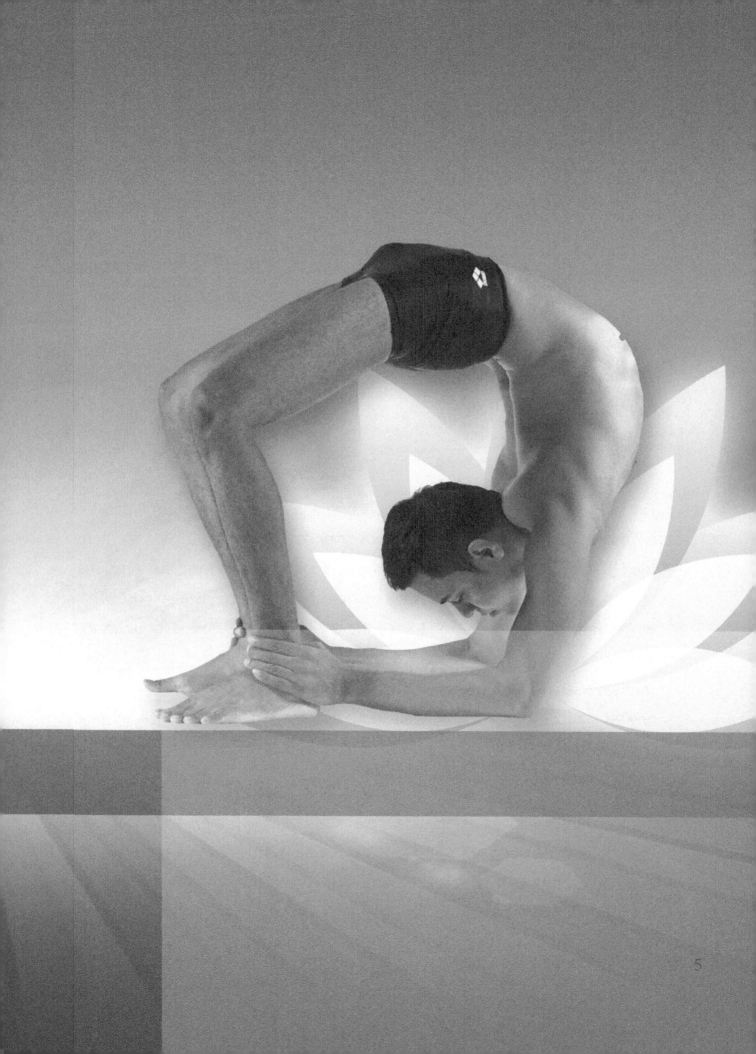

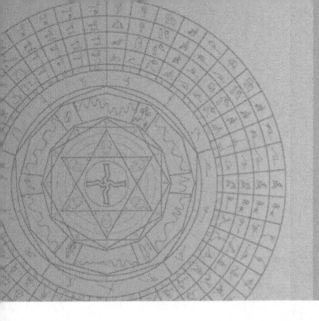

INTRODUCTION OF YOGA

Upanishads;

We are what our deep diving is,

As our desire, so is our will,

As is our will, so is our act,

As is our act, so is our destiny.

Our body is made out of a complex phenomena. Researchers are still dazzled by its sophisticated functions. Modern science is coming up with so many hypothesises about the beginning of our evolution and its incredible functions, yet researchers present their results as though they come as a surprise. That which modern science only now sees, the ancient sages encoded for us on the internal level long ago. Here the East and the West are getting closer and closer through science, but ancient yogis never looked at this planet with the idea of any separation. Their works were all about the function of this massive universe and how that massive universe helps us to realize itself through us. That is the beginning of what this yogic journey is about.

The cosmos is a composition of five elements: akasha (ether), vayu (air), agni (fire), apas (water), and prithvi (earth). As inhabitants of a physical body, we are composed of these five elements, about 70 percent being water. The human body is a complex, sophisticated system created by the universal cosmic intelligence. Whatever we are seeking with the help of science is nothing but the primitive version of what the universe has already given to us. While we try to change and modify what we know by learning from this planet, we must see that there is nothing new that can be done from this human perspective.

Ancient India birthed an immense potential to realize the path of liberation, and yet, right now, it is hard for us to liberate ourselves from this very body. According to science today, in order to be liberated we must die. Yet because of its vast wealth and richness, the ancients of India discovered the path of enlightenment approximately 10,000-12,000 years ago. They provided the guideline for this path very clearly. Because of their insight and deep satisfaction with life, they did not seek the path of liberation out of irresistible impulse, but out of a conscious choice to understand the beauty of our fine being. Their whole approach is based on the idea of escaping the karmic cycle of death and rebirth in order to be liberated from the past and the future.

During the Vedic period, the highest action was dharma (intrinsic quality). One who harms no one but instead helps others is one who has the ultimate quality of action that one can share with other human beings. The path of liberation does not stop there. The idea of liberation spread throughout the countryside; it moved to Asia, and then around the world. Right now, yoga has gained more popularity around the world then in India itself, but the physical form of yoga alone is not going to make a human being more transcendent. We must instead embrace the classical way of how yoga was taught. We must each approach the right guru to help ourselves evolve and achieve a state of inner evolution.

The modern-day lifestyle is so rich. We have everything. Because of our more comfortable lifestyle, we therefore desire more and have more passion towards the external, material life. It has become a social status to have things that impress others and to show that our personal lifestyle is superior to others. This comparison creates misery, and in the heat of comparison comes worry. If someone is happier than us, we can't digest this idea. Therefore we try to improve by building bigger houses, but this still doesn't help us attain happiness. We can never reach a state of ecstasy because the point where we begin is fundamentally inappropriate. Because of the unclear mind, we repeat the past into this present moment again and again, and yet our suffering is never diminished. We still hope for the holy grail or another Christ to visit on this planet.

Our mind has become a dominant force towards an addiction to the memory of survival mode. For thousands of years, people lived in the trees, hid under rocks, and lived in caves. Man still holds on to that survival mode in the form of backstabbing, anger, jealousy, molestation, and betrayal. These have all increased among humans. Today, man's worst enemy is none other than himself. Sadly, nature's worst enemy is also man. The direction of the mind often leads toward destruction, not for life creation.

A small percentage of people live life joyfully with complete contentment. They live without repentance, but that is not enough. We are not here to destroy this planet which gave us life. We are here to bring a communion, a way to bring peace. Therefore, yoga is essential to make each human life more peaceful. We must create a healthy environment for this generation as well as the upcoming generations. The ancient yogis designed and created all the formulas needed to embrace and enrich life to its fullest possibility. It is completely in our hands to continue to change and to act wisely. Right action alone can bring total ecstasy in life.

This book will briefly guide your understanding of the core concept of yoga and spirituality. While some words might sound different, they belong to the same path. In my own life experience, when I began my practice at the age of twelve, I had no idea about spirituality. Although I was born into a Hindu family and yoga existed in the very tradition of Hinduism itself, one does not learn yoga just by doing something. Rather, the very lifestyle of the family was deeply embedded with the core concepts of yoga. We learned yoga incidentally and unconsciously.

Before I joined a yoga ashram, I was already reading and practicing from the book *"Light on Yoga"* by B.K.S. Iyengar, as he was my main source of inspiration to do asanas (postures). When I first joined the yoga ashram under the guidance of Yogacharya B. Dhinagaran, a disciple of Swami Gitananda Giri Guru Maharaj, I was already able to do a headstand. I was thinking that what I performed was already an advanced stage of physical yoga. I thought that my asana practice was better than that of others. With that in mind, at the moment I entered the yoga ashram, I was terrified to see that kids my age were already performing all of the hardcore asanas with ease and comfort. Their abilities were remarkable, with strong powerful backbends and handstands without any difficulty. By comparison, my ability was only up to the mark of doing a shaky headstand! Literally, I was threatened.

Later, when I spoke to those students about their amazing abilities, all they said was to practice regularly. They invited me to join in their practice sessions. Groups were divided according to ability. Among them were kids who were very advanced, and that fed my ego so well. Along with the crazy asanas, we had to perform karma yoga (selfless service). That was mandatory in the southern part of India. At that young age, we enjoyed performing karma yoga regularly. After my school hours, I went directly to the yoga ashram to learn the asana (postures) and to hear the simple discourses conducted by my teachers. I primarily resonated with my asana practice and was totally unaware of the spiritual level of yoga practice. Nevertheless, I was still fascinated and attempted to achieve the physical form of yoga practice more than any other sports.

In the beginning when I practiced yoga, it was all about doing asanas. With my beloved teacher, we traveled to participate in asana competitions in different cities around India. The more I participated in the competitions, the more I realized how weak I was. The regular practice and dedication helped me achieve the target I wanted to reach. While I was preparing for my graduation, my teacher also encouraged me to teach asanas and pranayamas to other students. That opened the door for me. For the first time, I was so satisfied with the class that I taught (even though it was a simple one-to-one session). To me, the joy of teaching was amazing! I give all credit and merit to my teacher, who encouraged me constantly to teach for six years in India.

I was uncertain about my future. Due to my family's poverty, my family wanted me to choose the work that would make money. They did not want me to choose yoga. Our culture is not like in the West. Once you graduate you are not simply free to choose your profession according to your personal wishes. As an Indian, I was expected to provide for the care of my family. Yet, I felt some sort of emptiness lurking within me as my suffering was not reduced any further.

On the day that I won several prizes, I was on top of the world; but later, the mind came into play and made me restless, agitated, and muddled. I understood that I had an emotional weakness but was yet unaware that the key, the solution, was within me. I had no idea what to choose as my profession. At the same time, my graduation was coming. Eventually, I chose to work in the corporate industry. I worked for a year right after my graduation, but still I felt unsatisfied. As my practice had become less, my body became weaker and I literally had to give up asana practice. During that moment my elder brother, Gopal Krishnan, who was working in Hong Kong, gave me an opportunity to restart my yoga career. The moment I heard that news, I literally abandoned the corporate industry.

Still with a lot questions in my head, I started to work in the fitness industry. I enjoyed teaching yoga in Thailand, but my own misery had not come to an end. My emotions bubbled up many times during those years. In 2008, I went back to

India to attend a meditation camp for one month in a reputable center. For the first time, I was able to unravel the knots between my body and my mind. Those strong meditation tools worked inside me like a miracle. The very essence inside me had changed. Since then, yoga is no longer an asana practice but a way to manage my lifestyle. It was the gateway for me to grow further.

In my childhood, all I knew was to wake up early and practice yoga relentlessly. Once I did the meditation camp, I became interested in knowing my true self, and silence. With that interest, I was able to see my surroundings more peacefully and with tranquility. Since then, meditation has become a strong part of my life. When I teach yoga for many hours in a row, which can be very draining, all I need to do to restore my energy is to practice the meditations I learned in India.

As the years passed, I worked in Singapore, but I came back to Thailand to open a place where I could teach yoga, as authentic yoga. Since then, my passion for yoga has expanded. In the meantime, I met my Universal Yoga® teacher - Andrey Lappa. He is as powerful as a lion and as soft as an innocent child. When I studied with him, his teachings immediately resonated with me. His experience is so vast. He has travelled and studied in India more than 40 times and in Nepal almost 40 times. With such experience, he created his own unique system called Universal Yoga®. It is not a different style of yoga, please don't misunderstand here. His teachings fully belong to the Vedic system of yoga and to the Tantric tradition. The very name "Universal Yoga®" can look unusual for many Indian people. In the West, yoga is often too general and narrow. And many western people simply don't understand if someone calls yoga as simply yoga. Everyone wants a second word, to name, label, and then market as a specific method by a particular teacher. That is why, when teaching yoga programs to western students, Andrey was pushed to add a second name to the word Yoga (at the beginning he was always teaching using only the single name Yoga, as it is used in India). By adding the word Universal, he wanted to point out to the western students that he is teaching not some narrow specialized method of yoga, but all the traditional system of yoga as it is, including the methods and practices for all of the human shells: physical, energetic, psychic, mental, and karmic. What Andrey Lappa teaches under the name Universal Yoga® is traditional yoga.

If you dive deeply into his teachings, you will understand that it is not just a style of practice, but rather a way of consciously living a yogic life. His teachings are all about how to raise your frequency of awareness to the next level. His experience and teachings will surely make any serious practitioner dive deeply into yoga. His intellect and the clarity of his vision is amazing. His research in the field of yoga shows his passion and curiosity. He has dedicated his whole life for the sake of yoga. He is not only an inspiration, but a Master who can influence your body, mind, and spirit. His very presence will raise your awareness, in the same way that we gain awareness by meditating. His research in asana, vinyasa, and sequencing is brilliant. He is the first person in the field of yoga to discover, unlock, and organize a comprehensive system for the creation of unique asanas. Andrey

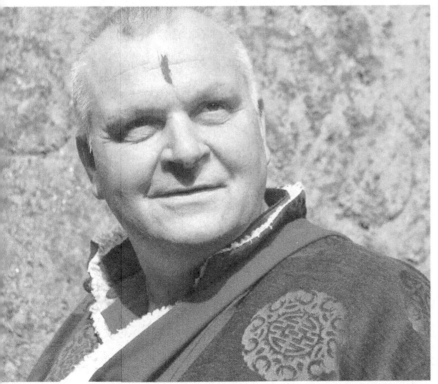

uses his creativity of asanas, plus the full system of Himalayan vinyasa, and combines that with profound sequencing methods to allow the practitioner the opportunity to reach samadhi through a physical practice. He is a Master of creative asanas, vinyasas, pranayamas, and Shiva Nata® (Dance of Shiva®). In order to learn more, go through his book called Yoga: Tradition of Unification.

Andrey Lappa

With his phenomenal innovations, he has designed the 4x4 Universal Yoga® Mandala sequence of asanas, vinyasas, and pranayamas that I describe and demonstrate in this book. This is only a fraction of the information about Universal Yoga®, yet I hope it would be an inspiration for the seekers to get the ultimate bliss from yoga.

In this sequence you have access to both "Ha" and "Tha" based asana practices. The word "Ha" refers to the strengthening asanas and the word "Tha" refers to the stretching-based asanas. All of these methods are crafted systematically to ensure that throughout the practice, you are fully conscious and doing postures that touch all of the marma points in your body, without injury.

Traditionally, yoga practice is done facing one side only, East. But there are many prayers and offerings traditionally used for the four sides of the world in Hindu and Buddhist yoga practices. Andrey's insight is amazing and logical. He emphasizes that we must face all directions during practice. To understand and decode this practice, one must be firmly established in the field of asanas, vinyasas, pranayamas, and meditation. It is an ideally balanced sequence that allows your body and mind to increase its range of awareness. On another level, the vinyasas with turns in every direction will blow chaotic thoughts away and will create energy and mind balance. Go through Chapter 1 - Chapter 7 to understand the core concepts of asanas, vinyasas, pranayamas, then learn the 4 x 4 Universal Yoga® Mandala sequence in Chapter 8. The last two chapters explain some of the practices in greater detail.

Namaste

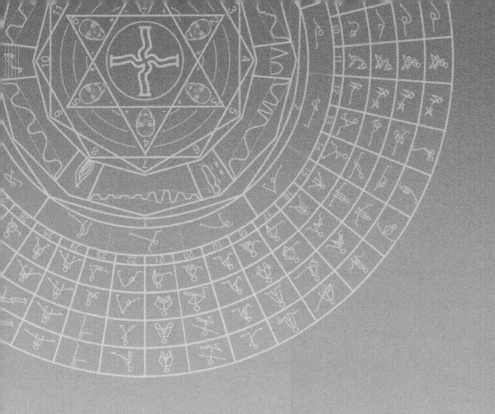

CHAPTER 1

What is Universal Yoga®

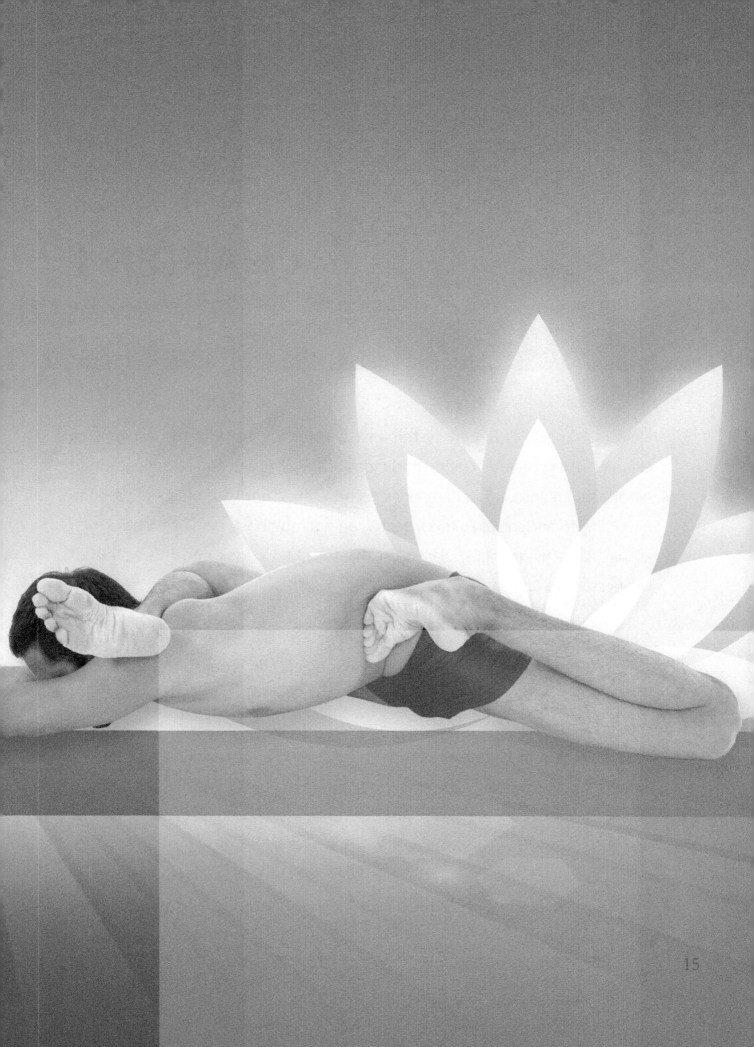

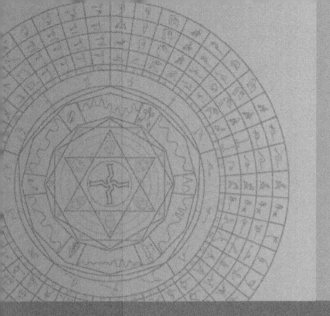

CHAPTER 1

What is Universal Yoga®

Universal Yoga® is a well systematized approach leading the aspirant to experience a completely different dimension of physical, energetic, mental, and emotional balance. It is cutting-edge technology strung with pearls of wisdom. According to ancient yogic texts, each man is a multibody being who has seven koshas (sheaths or shells). Based on this topic, let's look into the system of Universal Yoga®.

A human being consists of seven layers within the body. Yoga is the methodology through which to understand and direct our practice in order to create balance on each shell, between the shells, and between the individual's shells and surrounding space. Many schools emphasize only the physical body. Some schools insist on just pranayama. Some schools emphasize mainly concentration. Other schools emphasize more asana and less pranayama and meditation, or vice versa. Each of these types of practices are classified and practiced according to one's own karmic motivation. It is not wrong to practice asana alone. For instance, youngsters are more energetic, if you ask them to sit calmly and silently, they will literally experience chaos in their minds. Therefore, asana practice can be a great tool to activate the body. After an asana practice you can ask children to sit still for a while. Physical and mental activity is needed prior to encountering stillness.

If an adult's body is weak and ill, asana is a great aid to regain health. Similarly, a person with mental issues must utilize yogic techniques involving concentration and visualization because just doing an asana practice will not be of great help.

The different facets of yoga technology vary from person to person, and the amount of interest you have will guide you to begin establishing that particular field of interest. The practice of yoga can change a poor lifestyle into a healthy one. You can let go of old habits and cultivate new healthy patterns in your life. When you are weak and ill, your body will not have the capacity to achieve the final result. The same is true if you have poor concentration or poor memory; you can say you are dragging in this life. Literally, it becomes a spiritless life. Adding spiritual strength to life is one of the main targets of the vedic system.

If yoga is practiced by targeting only the body, physical alignments, or how many poses you achieve, then you will be able to look back and see how much you have improved on the physical level. Specifically, physical practice is effective when you learn from an educated teacher who knows how to adjust your body and lets you know how to improve your asana skills in a safe way. Yoga doesn't, however, end there. Rather, you must perpetuate the other aspects of yoga into your daily practice. This can help your mind to be calm. Your emotions then will not let you become distracted. You will gain a level of energy to prepare yourself for your own inner transformation.

In the beginning it is perfectly fine to practice asana, but later you must learn how to spend more time for your internal practice as well. I am not trying to say that you should stop asana practice and focus on your mental practice alone. It is just that I have seen teachers talk about inner transformation and they act as if the body is the enemy, and they have no physical discipline over their own body.

In Universal Yoga®, we are not against the body. The body is primitive, yes. The yoga process ultimately helps us understand the mechanism of the mind but connecting with the body is the first step in this process. This first step helps you understand the bioenergy of your subtle system. Through physical practice, you will know that your body and mind are filled with intellect, because each thought is powerful even if directed toward the body. This process can change and shift your energy depending on your thought process. If you have accumulated toxins in your mind through emotional traumas, negative relationships, frustrations, negative discriminations, and wrong judgments, then your mental impressions will totally disconnect you from reality. But, when you know how to bring alignment within these layers, and you learn how to eliminate impurities from your inner system, your level of energy becomes high, and that is when the true journey of enlightenment begins. Therefore, in the system of Universal Yoga®, you must practice and work on each shell. Unless there is one single practice that can be accorded to all the shells, you cannot progress without a push and pull. Should you truly want to break free of the clutches of your body and mind, only raising the consciousness will help you attain the goal of yogic perfection.

My teacher, Andrey, has created a unique system which is helpful in finding balance within each and every shell respectively.

The Seven Koshas:

The word "kosha" mean sheaths or shells. And the word "maya" means illusion. The Vedic *Upanishads* have explained that the body consists of five shells. Later, other *Upanishads* mention the koshas having seven layers. In this context, we refer to the seven shells. As each shell represents our superficial layer to the inner core, so you first develop each shell individually, and later you create balance between the shells. At the third stage of practice, you find balance between the shells and the surrounding atmosphere.

We call each layer "maya". It is said that the very body you look upon is not reality. Everything is in a state of constant flux, we do not know whether it is a dream or reality. Today the science of quantum physics concludes the same. What we see is nothing but an illusion. For example, the body is not yours as you think. Nor is the mind. This is also so with the Self. The interesting thing is that the Self is not yours because it cannot be possessed. It is easy to say that it is infinite, but let's analyze that which you call yours. At night we dream, and the moment we are awake the dream figure and the conversation that we had in the dream is gone. Once you are awake, the dream becomes unreal; yet in the day, we also dream. When you go to sleep again, the day has become a dream and the night has become reality. What is changing constantly is an illusion. The moment you raise your frequency of awareness to a higher level is what we call "reality". Reality is when you know that you are not the body or mind but an everlasting phenomenon. The very witness is what we, in the East, call 'reality'. It is apart from all else that we experience. Life is nothing but the projection of the unreal world.

Now let's briefly look into the seven layers.

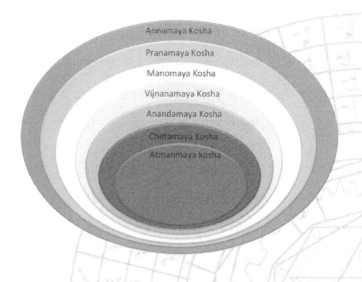

Figure 1:1

Anna Maya Kosha: is the food body, a gross and more superficial layer. You become what you eat. Here, food becomes your body. It is composed of flesh, blood, and bones. It is a solid substance that identifies with the planet on which we live. This first layer is like the hardware of a computer, the physical shell.

Prana Maya Kosha: is the energetic body, body of sensation. Sensation can happen in many ways. It may be through pain or pleasure. This layer is connected to the subtle level of the body.

Mano Maya Kosha: is the mental body (manas, chitta), filled with mental impulses. This layer relates to the psychic shell.

Vijnana Maya Kosha: is the supramental body, wisdom and higher intellect generated in the mind. It is an intellectual layer; yet it is an illusion of the intellectual layer that you are intellect.

Ananda Maya Kosha: is the etheric body, or blissful body. When one dives deep into one's nature, one experiences everything as bliss. It does not happen from outside. The quality of bliss cannot be destroyed by any external circumstances. It flourishes as a result of one's true nature. If you are in total reality, you are nothing but full of bliss.

Chitta Maya Kosha: in this layer, one has neither misery, nor does one crave for bliss. One goes beyond thoughts. Still, this step is fragile. It has all the possibilities to fall short because the samskaras (latent impressions) are not completely destroyed here. There is still the desire to be alive on this planet.

Atma Maya Kosha: atma is a complex of karmic motivations, depending upon one's lifestyle. If the lifestyle is not in symmetry with the karmic motivations, then everything around us will be a mess. This shell reflects the deep root of our character and who we are. If your motivation in life is matched to your dharma, then your actions reflect your state of consciousness. The reverse is also true. If you live a life of suffering and have deep inner turmoil, this is also reflected by your actions. The aim of yoga practice is to change the very core of misalignment that we created within ourselves through any wrong habits or wrong lifestyle choices. As you realize and progress toward the path of dharma, then you can craft a symmetrical state of balance that will lead you towards the path of moksha (liberation).

It is good to analyze the weaknesses in oneself, but how does one overcome them? What are the techniques needed to practice and build a shield against all odds? Here, Patanjali has given us two strong keys to direct our mind to achieve the desired result as well as help us to travel into the journey of yoga without any misdirection.

Yoga Sutras of Patanjali (Chapter 1.12):

abhyasa vairagyabhyam tannirodhah

- abhyasa: constant or repeated practice
- vairagyabhyam: non-attachment, neither attraction nor aversion.
- tan: of those, through that of
- nirodhah: cessation, control, restrain, integration, coordination, stillness

Abhyasa and Vairagya (Keys to Success):

Emotions are neither negative nor positive. How one travels through the world using the five organs of perception must be analyzed carefully. Ordinarily, you can see that many people live in constant states of anger and sadness, and can be easily provoked. In fact, many people are already angry before a situation happens. Then no matter the situation, they feel justified showing a negative reaction. Based on this, people can sow many seeds of emotional bondage.

Yogic rules were developed mainly to liberate oneself from these emotions such as fear, anger, greed, lust, jealousy, attention seeking, possessiveness, and depression. When these calamities hit our inner world unconsciously, our bio-rhythms begin reacting. It is as if one has thrown a big stone into a clear pond of water. These changes are not under our control. If it is needed, it will come. If it wants to, it can leave anytime. As a result, we end up not only messing with ourselves but also with the circle of those with whom we relate. These causes and effects become inevitable to an untrained mind. Yoga mainly emphasizes the need to create a new pattern to stop all these emotional calamities. It occurs through regular abhyasa (constant inner practice) and vairagya (detachment). Regular practice is the medicine for these emotions. Vairagya (detachment) helps one from repeating the past. It doesn't mean you have to stop all of your desires. These methods are mainly given to break the accumulation of old habits. The mind can play a game here. Because constant practice with effort might make a seeker feel bored over time, detachment is necessary. Detachment helps make a practice effortless. It also helps cultivate new habits which eventually lead one to master the calamities of the mind. Or, as in Patanjali's description 'yoga chitta vritti nirodhaha', it helps stop fluctuations of the unstable mind. When you cultivate your practice through these two aspects, you become capable of dropping the old patterns which had been cultivated primarily through the five organs of perception (ears, eyes, nose, tongue, and skin).

Purusha and Prakriti:

Human suffering is caused mainly by ignorance. According to samkhya philosophy, the dual concept of purusha and prakriti plays a major role.

Purusha means consciousness, self, or seer. Prakriti means nature. In simplified terms, we can refer to purusha as the 'subject' and prakriti as the 'object'.

We can count the body and mind as part of prakriti, too. But the Self or the witnessing Self is purusha.

We use labels in our day-to-day life to identify objects, such as birth name, religion, category, country, educational qualification, emotions, successes, failures, gender, desire, and ego. These all belong to the object to which we are identified. Such labels constantly distract us away from purusha, which is a pure consciousness. This causes us to be mainly identified by those objects and thus entangled in the eternal web of suffering. We express objects with labels to understand the nature of our material life, but we can transform beyond that. This cycle of labeling and misidentifying with the object repeats constantly until we realize the nature of purusha, and who we truly are. Yoga can help with this understanding.

The samkhya system tried to convey these messages of understanding purusha, thousands of years ago. However, people are still entangled with desires and therefore experience pain in the external world. Suffering is a need that everyone must encounter on this planet, as an experience. But once the spirit is awake and one strives to attain the truth of what is real and what is just an illusion, then it is possible to end suffering. This is similar to the Buddhist approach. At the peak of awareness, consciousness can reflect like a mirror. If one understands the observer, the one who is observed or the one who can understand that the object does not belong to the spirit, then the path of inner revolution happens. The attainment of moksha (liberation) is possible in this lifetime.

Three Gunas:

Sattva: luminosity; rajas: activity; tamas: darkness.

In yogic philosophy, matter means prakriti. The five elements (earth, water, fire, air, and ether) are part of prakriti. There are also three states of gunas (fundamental qualities) manifested by prakriti. This idea is in the Vedic yogic tradition, *Yoga Sutras of Patanjali,* and the *Upanishads*.

The fundamental qualities or gunas refer to three different natures. This has been explained in detail in Ayurvedic teachings. Here we will just look at these categories briefly.

Sattva:

A state of calmness and cleanliness. The consciousness is in complete balance and we can experience this stage in life, either consciously or unconsciously. It is a state where the mind is not fluctuating. The mind is more peaceful and content. It is not arguing, nor is it pushed or pulled. We function from the higher qualities of the buddhi (intellect) which is a reflection of the true Self.

Rajas:

A state of movement. A dynamic lifestyle is hyper and always in a state of hastiness, never coming from a place of stability. It comes with changing plans frequently. It is an agitated and fickle state of mind. One is always identified by the mood of likes and dislikes. Emotions like jealousy and greed can anchor one down. One can be driven crazy by desires and wants. If you know how to channel and approach your desires carefully you will bring the quality of sattva inside and overcome rajas. On the other hand, if the strong desires overpower the sattvic nature,one becomes relentlessly entangled with the desires. Until the desires are satisfied, one cannot return back to the sattvic state.

Tamas:

A state of inertia. Here we experience that sometimes the mind is confused and unclear. We are stuck in the everlasting whirlpool of the mind. It pulls you very low and you experience heaviness, exhaustion and sluggishness. The mind will not allow you to understand the growth of the inward journey, or we can say the mind becomes delusional. It is an unclear state, as if the mirror of life is filled with dust, and it has to be cleaned in order to bring the awareness in. That awareness is the quality of sattva which one can use to overcome the state of tamas.

All these stages are constantly fluctuating in our lives. Obviously, one cannot be in one state all the time; rather you move from one state to another. That movement reflects our nature. When you do a regular asana practice you can see the fluctuations. Sometimes you feel so good and can do the whole class energetically; whereas on another day, you may feel tired, and you won't want to practice at all. This oscillation constantly happens not only while one does an asana practice but also in day-to-day life. Notice the constant change of your mood during daily activities.

By having a regular yoga sadhana and improving your diet, you can stop these constant changes of mood. In the yogic tradition, it is recommended to leave part of the stomach empty. It is a healthy way to maintain proper digestion and to absorb the proper nutrients. Here, one part of the stomach can be filled with solid food, one area is for water, and the remaining part should be empty. The empty state is more important to break up the food and help digest the food efficiently. It will lead to optimum health of your digestive system. Thus, you can build up the sattvic state and be more stable. Along with a better diet, regular asana practice is essential. In addition, a strong passion to attain the ultimate state is necessary. One's thinking should be more organized and stable as well. For example, if the alarm is set to wake you up at 5 am., but you hit the snooze many times, you may repent your own inability to wake up and that you wasted the morning practice in sleep. This oscillation must change. You must become ready to dedicate yourself to your practice. Dedication and readiness can lead to a quality of illumination, serenity, and peace.

Conquer Fear:

Fear is one of the major downfalls in any field. Fear happens when you cannot predict or when you encounter doubt! This happens to every individual. It is necessary to have some fear in our lives, and there is nothing wrong with that in general. But to experience fear in each and every step will make oneself feel small. Fear on the physical level is much more superficial than on the mental level. It is more challenging dealing with fear on the mental level. For example, handling an asana can be conquered through regular repetitions, but handling the fear of death is much more challenging. Yoga gives a step-by-step approach to overcome all emotional bondages. It helps set you free from all sorts of weaknesses of the body and mind. First, let's look into the physical aspects of fear.

Patanjali describes asana (posture) as the third step of the yoga path. Dealing with different kinds of asanas mainly helps you overcome physical weaknesses, but its primary function is to help you relax in a steady and comfortable zone during the practice. For example, an untamed man has every possibility to experience relaxation while sleeping or sitting on a couch and watching a movie. That is how he relates to relaxation. But it is quite different for the one who is awakened and can be relaxed despite any circumstance. This is what we call "a yogi" or "rishi"—the awakened one. This comes by simply understanding the body's nature. When the body is weak, it is very hard to be immobile and still. For example, if you feel dizzy, simply sitting on a comfortable bed will not make you feel completely relaxed. Even a small weakness can shake the foundation of the body. Imagine at the time of natural death, how much suffering the body has to go through! Therefore, yogis have found the method for overcoming this, by being still and immobile, but in a comfortable and relaxed state. The reasoning behind this is essential. As you train the body to be still for many hours, it is eventually within the body's capacity to remain still effortlessly. Therefore, yogic postures work as a great tool to tame the body. You are required to hold many different positions steady while keeping the mind in a relaxed state. This is healthy on the physical and mental level. These practices will lead the body to a capacity to sit steady for many hours. This is the perfect way to move onto the higher training forms of yoga.

On the mental level, fear plays a major role leading to sufferings such as stress, depression, anxiety, and insecurity. Fear can be the link that leads you further to other negative emotions, too, such as jealousy, anger, greed, hatred, and agitation. Dealing directly with the mind can be like a hide-and-seek game for the practitioner who has no understanding about the body-mind connection. Patanjali was a pure logical scientist on the inner level. His work made it possible for us to overcome these negative emotions.

If we understand emotions, we become closer to conquering fear. The major breakthrough happens only when we come to the state of "acceptance, awareness, and letting go". The main function of yoga is to delete all of the negative patterns from the mind, which in turn leads the body-mind complex to experience eternal freedom.

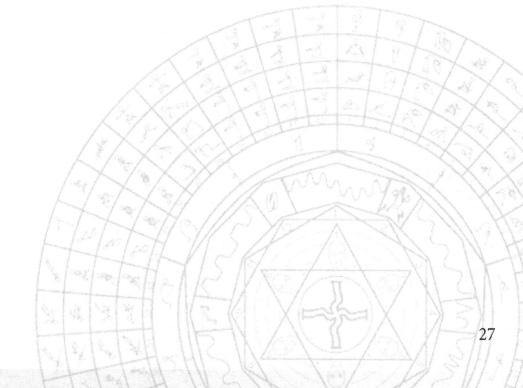

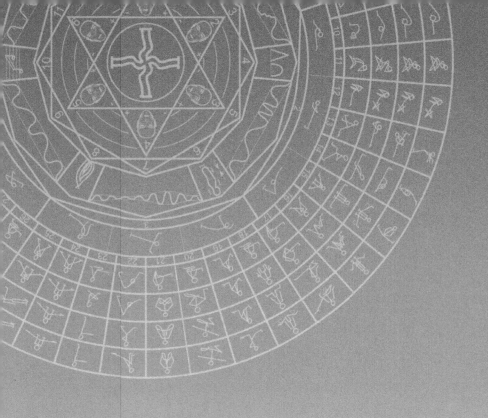

CHAPTER 2

Eight Classical Limbs of Ashtanga Yoga

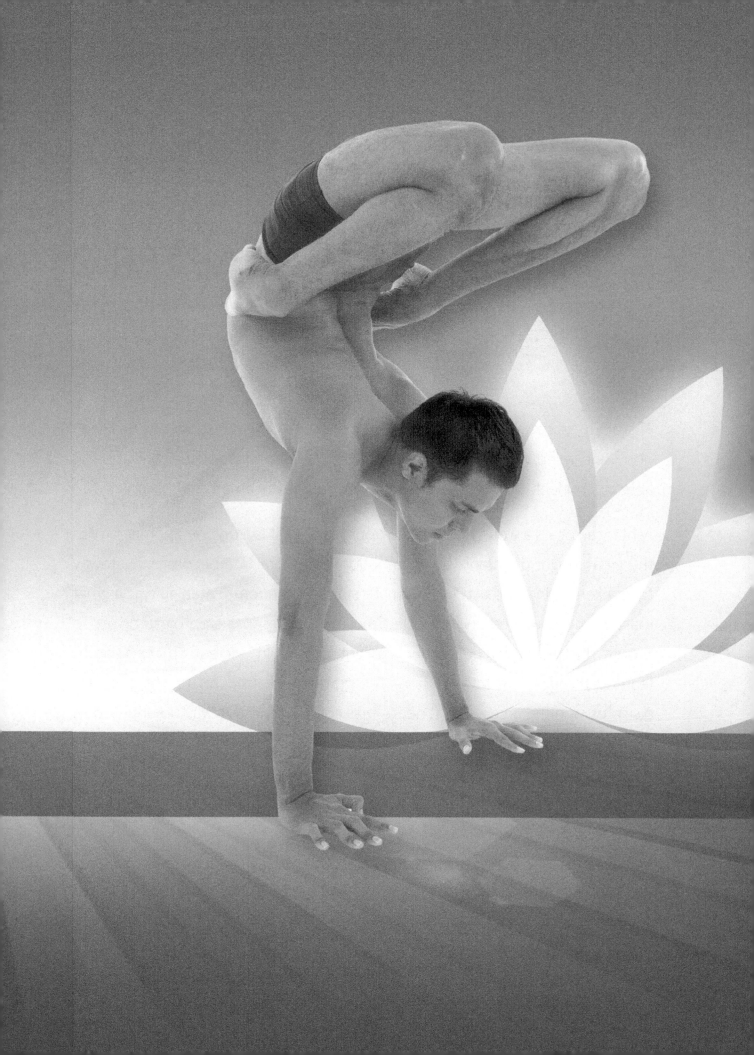

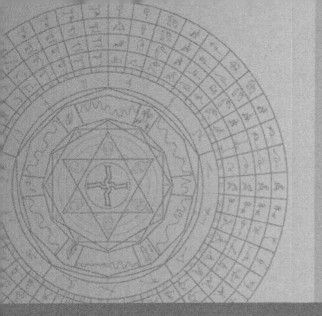

CHAPTER 2

Eight Classical Limbs of Ashtanga Yoga

The word "yoga" means to yoke, diversify, and unify. Creating harmony between body and mind with this unification, the individual consciousness (jivatma) is able to connect with the universal consciousness (paramathma).

Ashtanga Yoga is a well systematized approach, yet it is a unique approach. With the great insight of Patanjali's contributions, yoga practice becomes a gateway for seekers trying to reach the ultimate state of freedom. Patanjali was a great master who compiled and encoded these teachings in a step-by-step way to ensure that disciples could attain enlightenment. In ancient times, disciples learned through oral transmission. The guru transmitted his teachings to his disciples, and the parampara (lineage) has continued in this way up until today.

Once the understanding sprouts, the journey of yoga happens quickly. With sincerity, dedication, and devotion, it is possible to attain the state of kaivalya (liberation).

Here are the eight classical limbs (steps) of Ashtanga Yoga that Patanjali has defined in a systematic way. His yoga sutras can be a manual of study for all yoga practitioners around the world.

Yama:

Moral discipline. These rules are necessary when one enters the path of yoga. Without these patterns, practicing yoga creates chaos. It would be as if you would want to go right, left, up, and down all at once. It is impossible to go in many directions simultaneously. Therefore, it is necessary to follow these five steps:

1. Ahimsa: Non-violence
2. Satya: Truth
3. Asteya: Non-stealing
4. Brahmacharya: Chastity
5. Aparigraha: Non-greediness

Niyama:

Self-restraint. This is again about personal development. In order to progress along the path of yoga, these steps are essential.

Here, also, we have five main practices to begin with:

1. Saucha: Purity
2. Santosha: Contentment
3. Tapas: Self-discipline
4. Swadhyaya: Self-study
5. Ishvarapranidhana: Surrender to God

Asana:

Patanjali describes asanas as "sthira sukham asanam". Being steady and comfortable in the posture is very essential. Ancient yogis found that if you could understand this very body, you would have the capacity to understand the whole universe itself. Therefore, yogis have developed many asanas, from animals to birds and many other species. The main reason is because understanding the animalistic nature of yourself, or understanding your animalistic behavior, helps lead you toward a higher way of living. Through your practice you will be more capable of understanding yourself. Worldly desires will disappear naturally. It will not be done forcefully but out of one's own effort and sincere practice. It is sad to see the concept to yoga being reduced, in the West, to just doing the poses for the purpose of losing weight and getting fit. The essence of yoga in that approach is lost.

Now, western science incorporates yoga into therapy. Although yoga was not designed to cure one's physical problems, it can do that. Neither was it created in order to attain some physical benefits. Rather, yoga was meant to awaken one's highest potential possible. Unfortunately, people are often stuck and end up doing only the postures (asanas) not realizing there is more to yoga. It is as if one is sick and desperately needs some pills to cure the sickness and when one is not sick the medicine is forgotten.

Asana is not just a medicine to cure the aliment; rather, it is a bridge to move into the higher realms. Yoga embraces everything about what is good for humanity. While many have benefited from the therapeutic forms of yoga, real yoga doesn't stop there. Asanas are a preparation to create a strong body. Only a strong and healthy body is ready for meditation. A body formed through yoga can reach the pinnacle of willpower in order to gain the ultimate source of life within.

Pranayama:

"Pra" means existence, "ana" means cells, and "ayama" means expansion or control of this force. Prana also means that which existed before anything was created. It is also the breath of life. A cosmic ocean of energy is all around us, and it travels in our body and mind as well. With pranayama, the main emphasis is to restore your breath and to train the body and mind to suspend the breath for a period of time. This will accelerate vital forces from within. Yogis play with these pranayama techniques to even overcome death. Pranayama means one has the ability to control the prana at will. Pranayama should be done right after the asana practice. In order to do pranayama, one must have the ability to be still in asana.

When the body is strong and prepared, a yogi can go deep into the pranayama practice that includes kumbhakas and bandhas. These can be practiced separately or together.

The main parts of breath:
- Puraka: incoming breath
- Rechaka: outgoing breath
- Kumbhaka: retention of inhale
- Shunyaka: retention of exhale

The last state or stage of pranayama practice is called:
- Kevala Kumbhaka: the ability to hold the breath without any conscious control

Prathyahara:

Sensory withdrawal. "Prathya" means turning inward, "ahara" means food. This limb is about how not to entertain one's senses and how to detach from the sensory stimulations. It is also a means to declutter and detach from the signals the mind sends through the channels of the senses. It is the main goal on the path of yoga. This step is very crucial for all seekers. One may be good in the limbs of asana and pranayama, but if the senses overpower you, it is easy to get distracted and then get defeated, and just that easily, one can fall from pranayama and asana also. Training the senses is like training a wild horse. If the horse is tamed and trained properly it will follow your orders. If you try to control the wild horse without training, you could end up with a serious injury or even death. Controlling the senses doesn't mean trying to prevent their uses or the need to follow some masochistic idea. Rather, it is a complete understanding about your mind because the mind can provoke the senses to fall onto the wrong path, which leads to anger, frustration, and despair just to avoid further damage. Patanjali urges us to withdraw the senses and move to the inner world. Once you master withdrawal of the senses, then your consciousness starts to evolve. It becomes centered.

In a famous story from the *Bhagavad Gita* (Chapter 2, Verse 58 and 59), Krishna uses the tortoise (kurma) to illustrate sense control: "One who is able to withdraw his senses from sense objects, as the tortoise draws its limbs within the shell, is firmly fixed in perfect consciousness."

Emotions are constantly in flux. That is why they are called emotions (e + motion + s). We understand emotions as the perception of the mind because the mind judges, criticizes, misconceives, and condemns. These negative reactions happen because of ignorance (avidya) and because of the limited range of awareness resulting when one is heavily anchored by these negative sources. If you bring in the fire of awareness, the darkness of the ego disappears indefinitely.

Dharana:

Concentration, steady attention, or undistracted focus. It is not a forced state of practice. Initially, it is hard to fix the mind for even a short while. As one starts to know the weaknesses of his own source, he can practice holding the attention steadily. For this, there are hundreds of techniques, but if one learns many techniques blindly, they will simply be ineffective. Therefore, first pick up the method that your teacher guides you to choose. Slowly, after you master the technique, you can choose your own. Maintain that for a minimum of nine months to see the fullest results. As one evolves in the path of dharana, you will see the clarity arise within you.

Dhyana:

A constant steady flow of awareness. This means the ability to be in a state of non-doing for a long period of time. It also means the ability to sit with no thinking. That is what we call dhyana.

Here the attention is not narrow. Rather, the range of awareness expands and one can be aware of the surrounding space and oneself or vice versa. The object of the mind dissolves and you are no longer trying to fix or focus the mind on one point. Every school should guide an aspirant up to dharana. Through a successful dharana practice, one can attain this state. Here all techniques dissolve and one can be in a constant divine presence.

Samadhi:

A state of assimilation or a state where one will not function from the ego or an individual mind but as a cosmic being. One has attained the state of Buddhahood or Christ-consciousness. Here Patanjali has organized the many steps of samadhi meticulously. Even in samadhi, it is possible to have some samskaras (impressions), hence the many steps. If the samadhi has some samskaras and one still comes back, he has not been in the samadhi state long enough. Patanjali created a few steps to attain the ultimate samadhi, as one never turns back from that. Even in normal samadhi, one lingers and hesitates to rejoin the outside world. Any fall can be certain. Therefore, Patanjali gives these steps to overcome all hurdles. Patanjali defines these states in his classification of the various stages of internal meditation.

In *Yoga Sutras of Patanjali,* Chapter 1:17-18, he refers to two basic categories of samadhi:

1. Sabija Samadhi: "sabija" means with seed.

Here Patanjali explains sabija as with support or seed, giving a way to engage the mind (chitta) where it is not completely free from karma. The seed can grow anytime just as a tree, but there is still a chance to fall backward. Within the mind, the inner desires of life are still clinging somewhere.

Patanjali divides Sabija Samadhi into four stages:
1) Savitarka (with doubt or conjecture)
2) Savichara (with reasoning or pondering): intuitive experience mixed with discrimination and guided intellect.
3) Ananda (with joy): inner intuitive experience identified by feeling chitta or joy by chitta or joy permeated feeling.
4) Asmita (with 'I-ness' or individuality): intuitive experience mixed with a pure sense of being an individual.

The second layer of Samadhi is known as Nirbija Samadhi:

2. Nirbija Samadhi: "nirbija" means without seed.

It is without seed. The chitta evolves completely. With this deep understanding comes the point where the sage will not look back into his life nor return back to this planet again. A deep gratitude towards the life is present, yet there is also a complete detachment to both life and death. In this state, one can be karmically free from all samskaras (impressions) and become a fully-fledged jivanmukta (enlightened one). Here the seeker is no longer seeking. All seeking has ceased. He has no desire to attain anything. He is indifferent to all dualities, as prakriti and purusha are no longer separate. He has attained the ultimate state of transcendence which is a state of kaivalya (liberation).

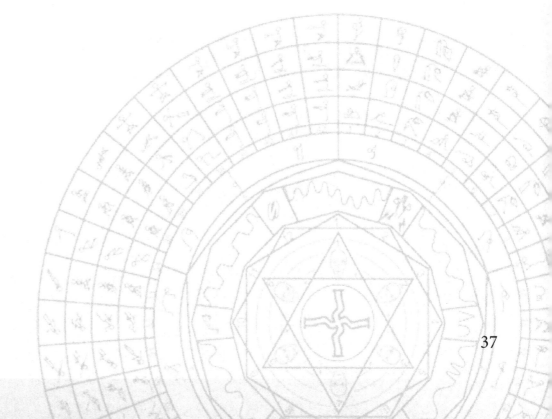

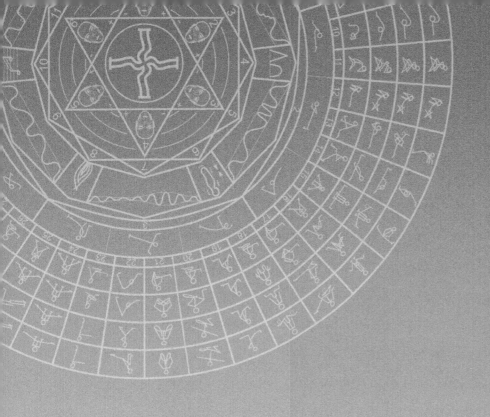

CHAPTER 3

Buddhism and Tantra

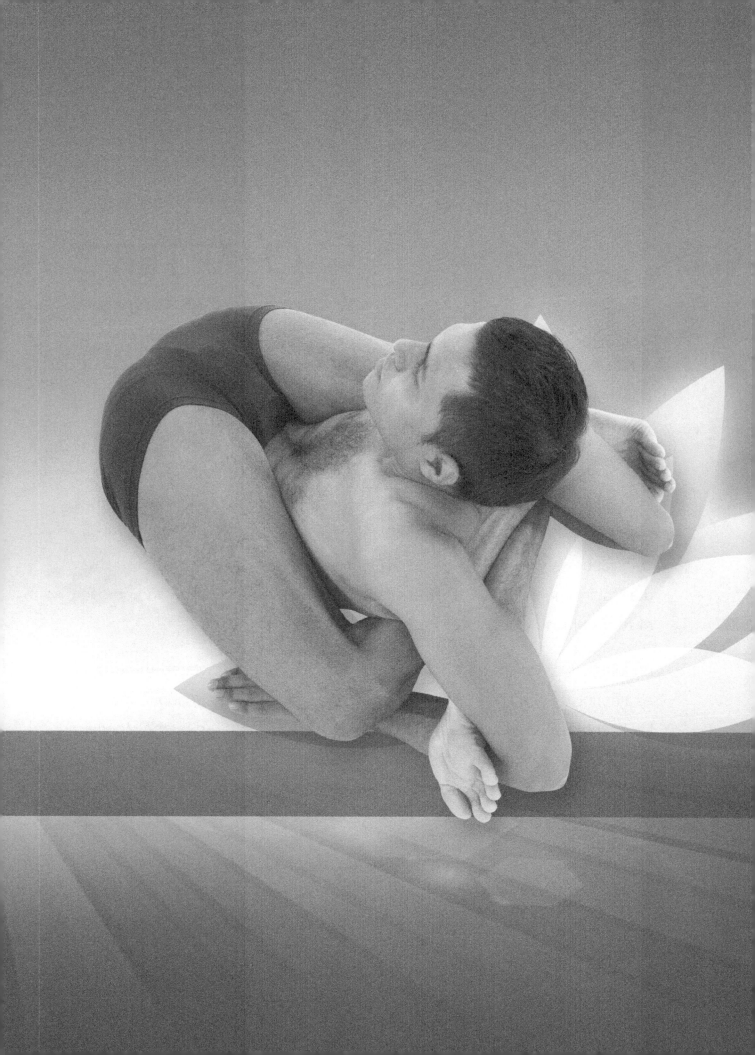

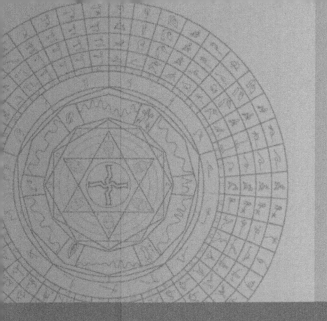

CHAPTER 3

Buddhism and Tantra

Sarvam dukham, sarvam anityam

All is pain, all is impermanent

Here Patanjali's and Buddha's approaches are similar. Both masters express their teachings in order to overcome suffering (that aspect alone is an extraordinary coincidence). Both schools have similar approaches and the aim is not to show that their school is better than the other but simply to illustrate an approach of the supraconscious state which goes beyond mind.

Buddhism blossomed on the Indian subcontinent and it travelled throughout Asia during the 9th and 10th centuries. Buddhist monasteries, schools, and their invaluable collections of books and libraries were demolished by the Mongols; however, the path continued to exist here and there. It was like an Olympic torch. Those ancient spiritual gurus lit the light, and it continued to burn in spite of the tough times.

Buddha's main emphasis was on how to train the desirous mind. Buddha realized that the source of physical and mental suffering began with the action of the mind. Thus, his main emphasis was to conquer anger through compassion and tolerance alone. It is through this path that one can reach the state of emancipation. The object of one's desire can change the direction of the destination, but it doesn't change the quality of life itself. The mind is always looking for the pursuit of happiness and comfort. The more we run towards happiness, the more we suffer because the very beginning itself is not the right starting point.

All of life's misery happens because of a lack of awareness. The activity of the mind is such that thoughts can travel as fast as the speed of light. So here, Buddha's approach was new and radical. He talked about ananda, the non-self. He neither accepted nor rejected the idea of God. He simply asked us to be in the middle. Although Buddha, the man, said nothing about God throughout his life, the man and his approach began to be praised as God in many countries in Asia.

It is easy to pray to Buddha as if he were God, but it is hard to walk in his footsteps. As in yoga, Buddhism emphasizes the path. The path is the key to unlocking the treasure within oneself. Patanjali mentions ishvarapranidhana as one of the important tools to attain a virtuous practice because a devotional attitude alone cannot attain the highest goal. Buddha, however, negated the idea of dualism because he was not satisfied with the greater ideas such as prakrita and purusha. Ideas alone cannot satisfy man's thirst for liberation. In fact, it can become a barricade to reaching nirvana. Buddha was not interested in divine theories. On the contrary, he was interested in the total effort, the dedicated involvement and the thirst for the truth to liberate the self (motivation). Knowing truth is a much easier path than understanding truth. Truth cannot be known dialectically; it must be apprehended through actual experience. Only then is it possible to transmute the flesh body into a divine body. That was the feat and reformation which Buddha had achieved. Once Buddha left his physical body, many theories started popping up. Eighteen schools arose around the first century BC. The first school was the Hinayana or small vehicle/cart. The second one was the Mahayana school, the great vehicle/cart. And the third school was Vajrayana, the diamond cart. In the diamond cart, the lower vehicle merges with the higher vehicle and they become one vehicle.

In the same way as Patanjali had his eight limbs path of Ashtanga Yoga, Buddha created the Noble Eightfold Path to overcome suffering based on his teachings. Let's look into this briefly.

The Noble Eightfold Path is:

- Right vision
- Right aims
- Right speech
- Right conduct
- Right livelihood
- Right exertion
- Right mindfulness
- Right unification

Buddha's approach was radical and was created towards liberation. Through his approach, thousands have awakened. His movement gained its greatest strength and dominance across Asia.

Tantra:

A revolutionary form of yoga

The term tantra comes from two roots: "tan" means to stretch or expand and "tra" means instrument. It is also said that tantra comes from two words: "tanoti" meaning to expand and "trayati" which means to liberate. Tantra basically means a technique that builds a new road beyond consciousness. It is a scientific and radical approach to go beyond the mind to attain the ultimate truth. It is not a philosophy to get the answer but an approach humanity can use to awaken from its deeply unconscious state.

Hatha yoga is a part of tantric methodology. In hatha we practice to cleanse the body, eliminate toxins, and remove all illness by practicing asanas, pranayamas, kriyas, mudras, and bandhas. In hatha we have the concept of sun and moon; similarly, the concept of Shiva and Shakti is more appropriate in tantra. Here Shiva is the consciousness and Shakti is the force. Here Shiva is sahasrara (7th chakra) and Shakti is muladhara (1st chakra). Here Shiva is ida nadi (left channel) and Shakti is pingala nadi (right channel). As a result, the dormant source of kundalini from muladhara is awakened and travels to sahasrara, and the nadi of sushumna (the central channel compared to ida and pingala) is awakened. In tantra, the energetic field comes into play. It is literally a union of Shiva and Shakti. Similarly, in yoga, we call this the union of the microcosm and the macrocosm. Unification happens and the state of samadhi or nirvana (ultimate bliss) is attained.

This is not a chapter that we finish here with hatha yoga. On the contrary, it is the beginning of yoga where the full tantric system starts to emerge. In India, the tantric movement has predominated for over 1,000 years, and it first appeared in the 4th century. Although it became notorious in the 6th and 7th centuries, it also became immensely popular during those periods. Tantra has borrowed from everybody, particularly from Samkhya and Vedanta.

Still this movement has an emphasis on strong sadhana (spiritual practice). For the first time in history, the feminine goddess entered into sadhana through the vehicle of tantra. Tantrikas give more importance to the female goddess while still emphasizing both the ideas of sun and moon and ida and pingala. Then rasas (emotions or moods evoked at your own will) come into play. Yantras (visualization methods) also predominate in the tantric movement.

Tantrikas do not emphasize the vedic languages, nor do they give more importance to Brahmanas. Their emphasis is more on the systematic approach by using the body as the vehicle for sensations and by stilling the mind through strong visualizations to achieve higher aspects of yoga.

Nagarjuna was a famous Buddhist philosopher who was adept in the Madhyamika system (middle path). He was also a comprehensible spokesman towards emptiness around the 2nd century. He was a native of Andhra Pradesh in South India from the Dravidian region. He was a famous and well-known master during the medieval period of Buddhism. Amongst other Buddhist schools, Vajrayana Buddhism evolved during the 4th century and gained dominance during the 7th and 8th centuries. Guhyasamaja Tantra is probably the earliest Vajrayana text. It is probably also the most important text.

Tantra's strong influence can also be seen in Kashmirian Shaivism as well as in the school of Trika. This system was first proposed by Abhinav Gupta. It reached its pinnacle in the 9th century. It was influenced by Saiva Siddhanta philosophy. This lineage invented 112 meditation methods (dharana practices) to reach the supraconsciousness and is very famous. It is said that Shiva himself is answering all of Devi's questions in the series of discourses outlined in this lineage.

Vajrayana Buddhism:

Diamond Vehicle

Vajrayana is mainly found in Tibet, Mongolia, the Himalayas, Ladakh, Himachal Pradesh, Sikkim, Nepal, and Bhutan. Vajrayana Buddhism is mainly popular in Tibet, and many Indian gurus travelled to Tibet and taught their lineages there. Whereas many Tibetans travelled to India and learned from many enlightened masters. People across the globe also came to study in Nalanda University, the location of one of the most renowned Buddhist schools in India. Despite the fact that Tibet is the powerhouse holding the Vajrayana tradition alive even now, many Tibetan schools have been demolished since the severe communist war erupted in 1949. Since that time, many Vajrayana teachers have been exiled and some have escaped to the heartland of India seeking refuge. Some of those very schools exist in Nepal as well.

This ancient yogic lineage contributes a lot to us. Among the many great siddhas of Vajrayana, Tilopa and Naropa were among the important masters to make the Vajrayana lineage more accomplished and successful. They believed in the systematic steps of practice that can lead one to enlightenment.

Here is a brief story about Naropa. In the 11th century a renowned Buddhist scholar, Naropa, was in search of a guru. As he traveled from India to Tibet, he was in search of many gurus, but he found none. Days passed. Weeks passed. Eventually years passed. Finally, he met an old beggar. At first, he did not realize that the beggar was his guru; but later, through his intense search he found the beggar to be his guru, Tilopa. He pleaded with the beggar to be his guru. Tilopa (the beggar) rejected him several times just as a means to test his will and his intensity. Eventually, the will, the interest, and the years-long sacrifices of Naropa led Tilopa to accept Naropa as his disciple. The years of instruction and practice passed and gave Naropa the fruit of complete self-realization.

This powerful system, which comes through strong ascetic disciplinary practices, gives seekers the trust that attainment of liberation is possible in this lifetime. Here practitioners accept the temporary negative concepts and emotions from their sources and transmute them into an enlightened being.

Vajrayana practitioners use visualizations as the main tools to reach the blank state of consciousness. Powerful visualizations help suspend one's flowing thoughts quickly. Then one can attain the higher state of consciousness or the state of "mahamudra" (the great seal or condition).

There are six major sects in this Tibetan tradition. They each convey the same message in a slightly different way. We will look into them briefly here. Right now there is enormous attention towards these schools; many books have been written extensively about these sectors.

Nyingma is one of the oldest schools in Tibetan Buddhism. It is also called the "red hat sect" founded by Padmasambhava, one of the most influential masters of Indian gurus.

Kagyupa is a school that promotes a yogic and highly ascetic method of practice. It has its roots in the tradition of the free yogis of the Himalayas and follows from the great masters Marpa, Tilopa, Naropa, and Milarepa. From there, it was transmitted to the Lord of Dharma Gampopa who monastacized the tradition. He is known as the main founder of the Kagyu lineage. The main emphasis of this lineage is to attain the state of kadampa and mahamudra, and it includes chakrasamvara and mahakala. They are known as "the black hats".

The **Sakhya** lineage is one of scholars or jnana yogis and was revealed by the Indian master Maha Yogivirupa in the 9th century. It was later transferred to the senior disciple, Khon Konchok Gyalpo. Sakhya teachings mainly emphasize Hevajra tantra, chakrasamvara, and mahakala. This is something that is common to both the Kagyu and Sakhya lineages.

Gelugpa is the youngest lineage. It is very popular for its emphasis on logic and debate. It was founded by the Tibetan master, Je Tsongkhapa Lobsang Drakpa. This school is known as "the yellow hats". The main teachings of the Gelug school came from the Indian guru, Atisha. Their focus is on attaining a state of supreme bliss and emptiness through compassion.

The **Jonang** school was founded in the 13th Century by Kunpang Tukje Tsondru.

Bonpo is a school of Tibetan Buddhism, but it has been called a non-Buddhist religious tradition that remained in Tibetan culture.

At the core of these lineages is the notion of yidams (deities), the spiritual guardians protecting and guiding those who worship them. Yidams, dakinis (enlightened feminine deities), and the Lamas (gurus and masters) are worshipped in addition to Buddha, Sangha, and Dharma which are known as the three roots. The ultimate refuge is the dharmakaya (truth/mind), sambhogakaya (energy/ speech) and nirmanakaya (physical/body) which are known as the three kayas or attainments. One who receives proper initiation from a lama in one of these lineages is able to access and reach the higher ascetic disciplines so as to turn inward thus beginning the journey on the path of enlightenment.

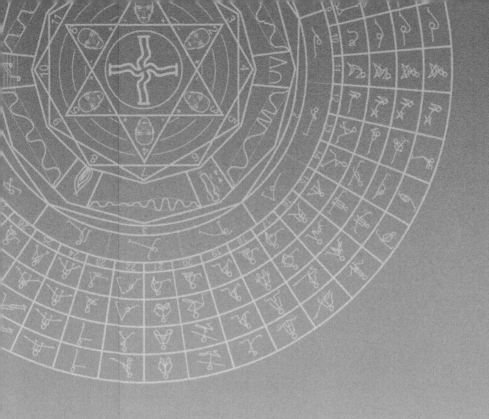

CHAPTER 4

Chakras, Siddhis, and Yantras

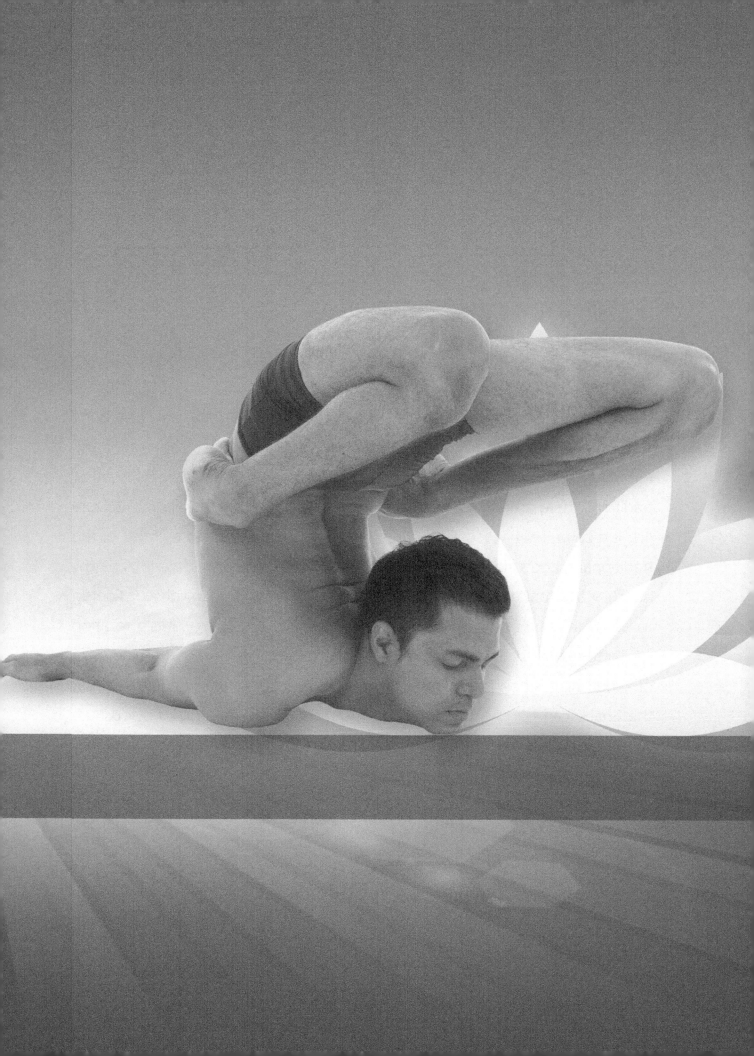

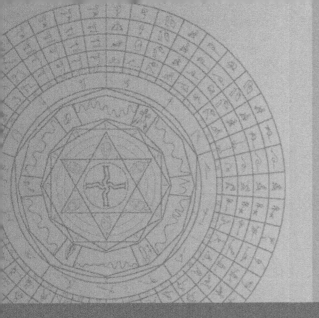

CHAPTER 4

Chakras, Siddhis, and Yantras

Chakras are energy centers. The vital energy of prana moves all over the body through channels we call nadis. The intersection where these nadis meet and form is a chakra. In some yoga traditions there are four chakras, while in other traditions there are eleven chakras. The seven shown in the diagram (Figure 4:1) is a commonly accepted number. This number is accepted by most of the traditional schools and lineages of yoga. Chakras can be imagined as either having a circular or a conical shape. In the vedic system chakras were mainly considered to be circles as that is what defines the rotation of the energy. It is a rotation similar to that of the planets and stars. This rotation therefore assists in the rising of kundalini. It is possible through yoga to rekindle the kundalini energy so that the Shakti can be awakened and transformed toward a supraconsciousness called Shiva. It is the state where Shakti meets Shiva. The awakening of this energy provides the surest way along the path of attaining the supreme state or enlightenment.

Look at the diagram (Figure 4:2) that shows the petals, elements, color, and symbols for each chakra.

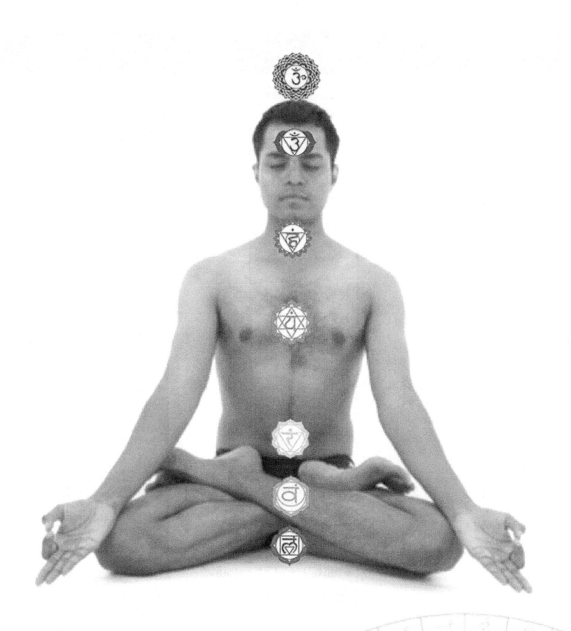

Figure 4:1

Chakra	Petals	Element	Color	Bija	Mandala	Rasa	Gland
Muladhara	4	Earth	Red	Lam	Square	Endurance, Biological Health, Lust	Coccygeal Plexus
Swadhistana	6	Water	Orange	Vam	Crescent	Playfulness, Sexuality	Sacral Plexus
Manipura	10	Fire	Yellow	Ram	Triangle	Will Power, Intention	Epigastric (Solar) Plexus
Anahata	12	Air	Green	Yam	Star	Compassion, Love	Cardiac Plexus
Vishuddha	16	Ether	Blue	Ham	Lotus	Intuition, Creativity	Laryngeal and Pharyngeal Plexus
Ajna	2	Mahat	Violet	Om	Infinite	Clarity, Rationalism, Logic	Cavernous Plexus
Sahasrara	1000	Space, Time	Pearl White	M-M	Boundless	Wisdom, Connection with the Supreme	Crown Center

Figure 4:2

1. Muladhara:

"Mula" means root or base. "Adhara" means support. This chakra is situated at the base of the spinal column between the anal orifice and genital organs, representing the element of earth. It has four red petals with the seed mantra "Lam" inside. It is also a seat of kundalini, where the serpent energy resides. This is the base chakra that should not be negated because the very foundation of life begins here. Overindulgence of food and sleep can block this chakra. Its symbol is an inverted triangle in the center of a square. Its vital breath is apana vayu.

2. Swadhisthana:

"Swa" means one's own. "Dhisthana" means one's own body. This chakra is situated in the spinal region above the genitals, representing the element of water. It has six lotus petals, with the seed mantra "Vam" inside. This chakra is a storehouse of all one's mental impressions that seek pleasure and crave food and sex. It has a white crescent moon and a dark sky as its symbol. Its vital breath is apana vayu.

3. Manipura:

"Mani" means gem or jewel, and "pur" means city. Usually, this chakra is called a "city of gems". It is situated in the middle of the spine right behind the navel. It can also be called the solar plexus, representing the element of fire. It has 10 lotus petals, with the bija mantra "Ram" inside. It reflects the life force and one's control of work. Its symbol is a red triangle, and within that triangle is a blazing sun radiating the energy of heat. Its vital breath is samana vayu.

4. Anahata:

This is the fourth chakra. The word "anahata" means unstruck or unbeaten. This chakra is situated at the region of the heart, representing the element of air. It has 12 lotus petals, with the seed mantra "Yam" inside. It is one of the most important chakras related to transforming the lower realm into the higher realm where loving kindness (metta) and compassion (karuna) start to flower. If one's anahata is awakened, that awakening is symbolized by the two interlaced triangles pointing in opposite directions. The upward pointing triangle represents the transformation toward the higher spiritual states and the downward pointing triangle represents one's understanding and awareness of the lower chakra states. Here it unifies and balances because one neither acts from the head nor is he stuck in his root center. Instead, a new transformation happens where he functions from the heart. One becomes the source of love and kindness. He becomes a compassionate being towards the whole universe. Its vital breath is prana vayu.

5. Vishuddha:

The word "vi" mean something great and unparalleled. "Shuddha" means beyond purity. This chakra can never become impure and hence never needs to be cleansed. It is articulated in the spinal column and medulla oblangata behind the throat. Vishuddha plays a major role in helping you discover your own unique self. It represents the element of ether (akasha) and has 16 lotus petals, with the seed mantra "Ham". It is a well-known fact that creativity is the strength of this chakra; one will be more creative and live life to the fullest extent. Life will no longer be boring or dull to him when vishuddha starts functioning. The mind is not a barrier but a vehicle used to transform oneself through creative ideas and thoughts. Hence it helps you become a unique being. One of the major drawbacks for vishuddha is having jealousy or comparing oneself, which can lead to great blockage of this chakra. It symbolizes the celestial moon-white elephant without a band. Its vital breath is udana vayu.

6. Ajna:

The word "ajna" means command. This is the command center which is also known as "chakra raj" the master of all centers. It is situated at the top of the spine, between the eyebrow center or the third eye. It lies in the region of the pineal gland connected to the pituitary gland (cavernous plexus). It has two lotus petals, with the bija mantra "OM" and is symbolized by the inverted moon and white triangle. You are no longer a protector of your own ego. The self is completely free where ida, pingala, and sushumna connect together. It is an awakened state where you are not functioning from the ego; you are functioning from cosmic intelligence. However, the chakra becomes blocked when one is serious about everything, or if one feels lost all of the time. Seriousness can close the mind pattern and cause havoc to the organism. Seriousness is a form of egoistic action where one disconnects from the cosmos. Yoga is mainly designed to eradicate suffering and accept the situation as it is. It is a language of communion with God. All methods of meditation are intended to accumulate strength and annihilate the function of the ego. One brings the light of understanding in and the darkness of ego dispels. Its vital breath is udana vayu.

7. Sahasrara:

This is the seventh chakra. The word "sahasrara" means thousand petals or brahmarandhra. It is the supreme experience of a thousand petalled lotus blooming on the crown. It is the meeting place of kundalini, where Shakti meets Shiva. The inverted lotus symbolizes the showering of the subtle body with cosmic rotations. It is also the center of the quintessential consciousness. By being in gratitude and not taking life for granted, one can enrich the flow of life to move in an upward direction. If one complains and is unhappy about what life has given, that itself can cause a blockage and tether one to the state of unconsciousness. Blossoming oneself is the ultimate gift that we receive from this cosmic intelligence. The attitude of being in gratitude is one of the most important messages that all yogis express in their own way. Its vital breath is udana vayu.

There is also vyana vayu which is circulating in all of the limbs and interconnecting all the chakras between themselves. Vyana vayu is responsible for the control of heat in our body as well as the energy balance between the chakras.

Nadis:

In Indian yogic language "nadis" means streams. It is where the subtle flow of energy moves like a river within these nervous patterns. In Chinese medicine nadis are referred to as "Chi" or the meridians. The yoga texts *Chudamani Upanishad* and *Yajnavalkya Samhita* describe that there are 72,000 nadis or bio-plasmic pathways. The *Shiva Samhita* mentions that 350,000 nadis emerge from the navel center, but there are 14 major nadis represented among them. Ida (left channel), pingala (right channel), and sushumna (central channel) are the most important nadis, and that is what Hatha yoga practices mainly emphasize for spiritual sadhana.

According to yogis, sushumna is the most important nadi. It is the gateway to attaining the higher realm of consciousness. Ida and pingala are the next two. The other 11 nadis are:

1. Gandhari: Extends from the edge of left eye corner to the big toe of the left foot
2. Hastijiva: Extends from the edge of right eye corner to the big toe of the right foot
3. Poosha: Extends from the left big toe to the right ear
4. Yashaswini: Extends from the right big toe to the left ear
5. Alambusha: Begins at the anal sphincter and ends in the mouth
6. Kuhu: Originates in the throat and ends in the genitals; as many say this is responsible for carrying seminal fluids
7. Shankhini: Originates in the throat and ends in the anus
8. Kurma: Originates in the anus and ends in the chest
9. Payaswini: Nadi that reaches the right ear
10. Shura: Nadi which sits between the eye brow
11. Vishvodri: Nadi that resides in the navel

Ida:

Ida relates to the parasympathetic nervous system. Ida nadi symbolizes feminine qualities, such as coolness, passivity, moon, and yin. The quality of ida is sattva, thus it creates a general state of relaxation in the muscles.

Pingala:

Pingala nadi relates to the sympathetic nervous system. Pingala symbolizes masculine qualities such as hot, dynamic, activity, sun, and yang. The quality of pingala is rajas. It thus releases adrenaline to activate the superficial muscles. It also helps deal with external activity such as stress, fear, and anxiety.

Sushumna:

Sushumna relates to the cerebro-spinal system. When the flow of energy is shifted to sushumna nadi, it symbolizes the quality of being in neutral. It is referred as "Brahman Nadi" because it is a state of brahman or a state of trance. One is totally established in the realm of awareness, and it is through this nadi that one can experience the awakening of kundalini.

Siddhis:

The word "siddhis" means occult powers. As is mentioned in many yogic texts, these powers are the natural outcome of the awakening of the kundalini. As one progresses, his practice and dedication are more for attainment of truth. Siddhis can happen. This is an indication that one is going on the right track, and that the track is not haphazard. It is a signal that shows that the way is right. Psychic powers may or may not happen. It is not our concern to play with them, but it is possible to make things accessible. Regular people may think it is impossible, but there are many psychic powers that yogis have accomplished.

Apart from yoga and tantra, siddhis can be achieved by past life experience. It is possible to bring the siddhis back into the present life. It is also possible when one is seriously injured or in the state of dying. In those states, one can express the siddhis. It is believed in India that through rituals and puja, siddhis can be awakened. It is possible to attain psychic forces through an intense yoga sadhana as well. There are many types of psychic awakenings. Some say that mahasiddhi is the most important one, more than all the other siddhis. There are many siddhis. Some writers say there are eight, others say 64, and some others even say 108. According to the *Yoga Sutras of Patanjali* there are eight main siddhis (ashta siddhis) which are the most important.

The Eight Main Siddhis (ashta siddhis) are:
1. Anima: One having the power of becoming minutely small like an atom.
2. Mahima: One having the power of becoming infinitely larger and greater.
3. Garima: One having the power of becoming infinitely heavy and immovable.
4. Laghima: One having the power of becoming totally light and weightless.
5. Prapti: One having the power of acquiring whatsoever he wishes.
6. Praakaamya: One having the power to be successful in whatsoever one desires. Having complete power of will.
7. Vashitva: Mastery to overpower others totally.
8. Ishitva: Realizing total supremacy or omnipotence.

Now modern science also has their own siddhis through gadgets and machines. Because of those objective materials, work has become faster and smoother. It is a way to get siddhis without conquering the I-maker which is the ahamkara. According to yogis, gaining siddhis does not mean one is awakened. The journey is not over yet. Rather, they are an indication to continue on the path meticulously.

Siddhis can be a trap if one is stuck there trying to prove his extraordinary skills to everyone because of an immature mind and inability to control the inner forces which he unleashed. Here the mind is still functioning and nothing much has changed. Diligent practice, with love and compassion alone, can help to attain the journey.

Mandala and Yantra:

Mandala is a geometric figure representing the universe and literally means "circle". They are complex matrix designs which may consist of of shapes like a square, circle, triangle, hexagram (star of David), or pentagon. In the center of a mandala there might be images of deities. A mandala can be drawn on paper, created with sand, on cloth, or with wood.

It was mentioned as early as the Rig Veda, but in Hinduism today, they call this "yantra". In Buddhism, such a design is called a "mandala". Every chakra is a yantra which has a bija mantra inscribed in it.

Mandala is a state of your consciousness when you draw a matrix symbol. It is not just a memorized picture. The way you draw it is coming from the state of supraconsciousness where the mind is not making any plan to design. Rather, the design happens spontaneously based on the vibrational expressions and understanding. Mandala represents the nature of the pure mind or no mind state. It helps to overcome distraction and creates a powerful sadhana that becomes an aid for meditation itself. It can be practiced by sitting in the middle of a mandala or by placing the mandala in front of you and fixing your concentration on it for a long period of time. Thus finally, one can reach the state of centeredness.

Yantras are used for magical reasons, to protect oneself (aksa yantra), to worship deities (devata yantra), and for visualization or meditation (dhyana yantra). Buddhist mandalas are used predominantly for meditation practices. In Universal Yoga®, the mandala or yantra is used mainly for visualizations and meditation. Yantras are also used for ritual purposes such as during a worship. In ancient days, yantras were used to worship certain deities. This was done to invite the deity and to achieve a desired result. According to Hindu tradition, a yantra is used for ritual and worship as well.

Samples of yantras:

Sri Yantra

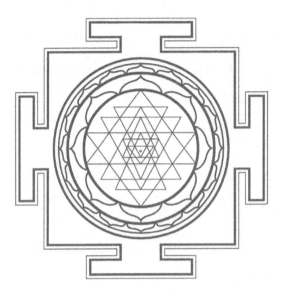

Figure: 4.3

The Sri Yantra is often referred to as the mother of all yantras. It contains nine interlocking triangles, surrounded by two circles of lotus petals. The image is framed by a geometrical gate called the "earth citadel". The nine interlocking triangles centered around the bindu (the central point of the yantra) are drawn by the superimposition of five downward pointing triangles, representing Shakti; the female principle and four upright triangles, representing Shiva; the male principle. The nine interlocking triangles form forty three small triangles each housing a presiding deity associated with particular aspects of existence.

Trika Yantra

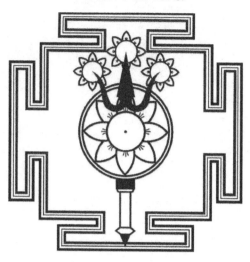

Figure: 4.4

The Trika Yantra represents the five powers of Shiva: consciousness, bliss, will, knowledge, and action. On top of the trident (Shiva's throne), sit three goddesses Para (divine will), Parapara (divine knowledge), and Apara (divine action).

Gayatri Yantra

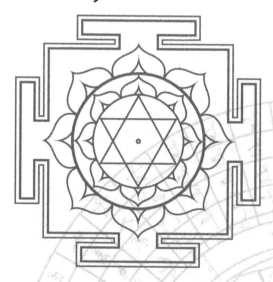

Figure: 4.5

The Gayatri Yantra is considered the most holy and auspicious yantra. It is used mainly for spiritual elevation. It represents the four Vedas and the fifth one represents almighty God.

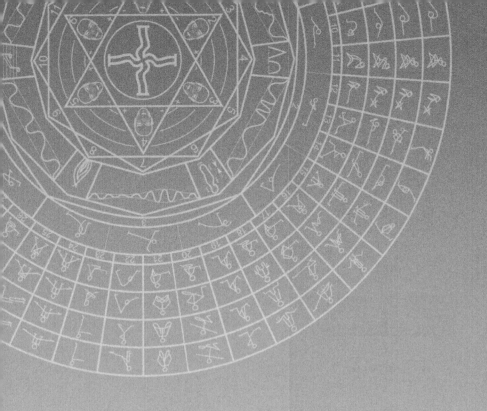

CHAPTER 5

Universal Yoga® Mandala

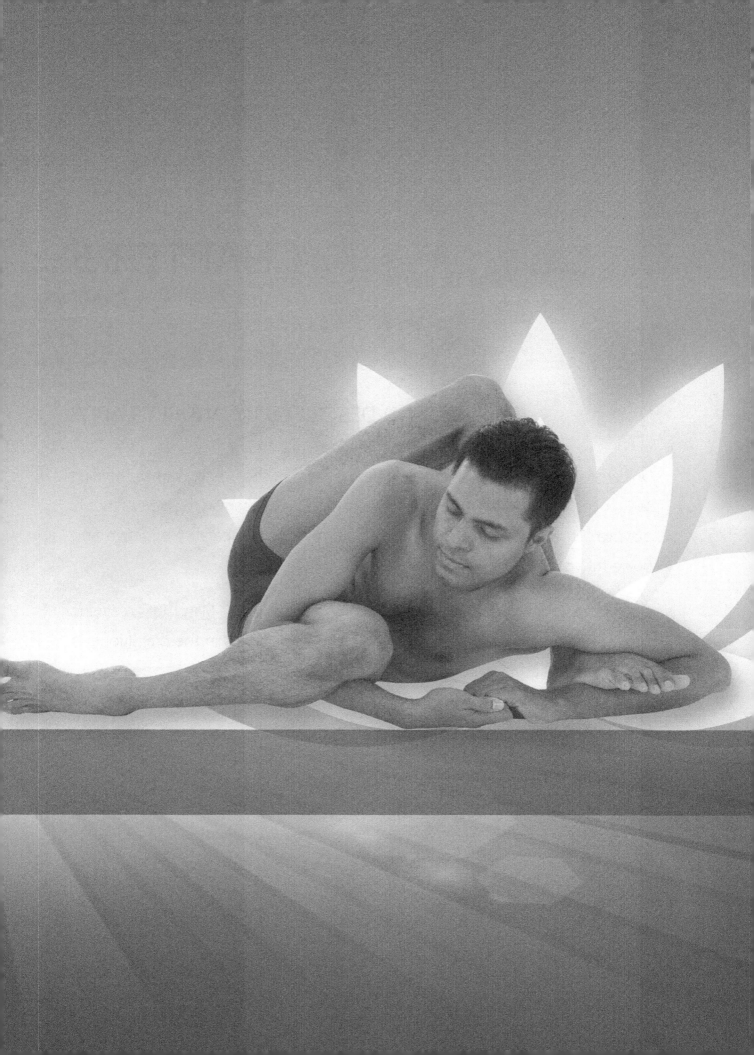

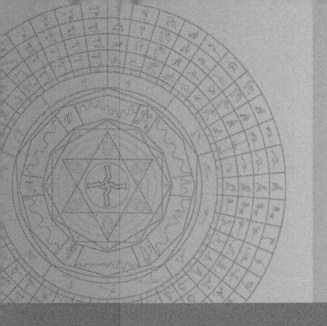

CHAPTER 5

Universal Yoga® Mandala

CREATED AND DESCRIBED BY ANDREY LAPPA

Universal Yoga® contains many unique asanas, vinyasas, pranayamas, training sequences, and yoga methods which are completely absent in the other schools of yoga. These attributes make Universal Yoga® a comparably effective and powerful yoga training system.

One of the unique methods represented in Universal Yoga® Mandala is reaching "chitta vrtti nirodha" (to not give birth to the fluctuations in the practitioner's consciousness) as a result of this unique practice.

This method is very important for all asana and vinyasa practitioners because it allows them to reach the authentic goals of Yoga utilizing the practice of asanas and vinyasas. Do not practice them just as Indian fitness, sports, or healing systems alone. Many other schools of yoga practice asanas and vinyasas just to gain health or lose weight.

For example:

1. Ability to develop the shape of asanas.
2. Ability to change the shape of the body for beauty.
3. Ability to improve the training system of stretching, strengthening, and body development.
4. Ability to cultivate the training for "yoga-sports" competitions only.

These external activities should not be identified as a Yogic destination. Unfortunately, such shallow goals are resulting in the majority of the yoga schools focusing on healing, Indian fitness, or yoga as a sport. Nothing is wrong with practicing healing, fitness, or sports; but they are not yoga, and they do not have the authentic yoga goals and methods. They replicate some ideas from yoga, but need to be called Ayurveda, Indian fitness, or another name — but not yoga.

Universal Yoga® gives its followers all of these results too, not as a main goal but as a secondary one, as "flowers on the side of the Main Path of Yoga".

The main point of the asana, vinyasa and pranayama practice is not the external forms or mastership of their techniques but their influence on the human sense of touch. Every asana, vinyasa, and pranayama produces specific internal feelings. This is a very important experience for every yoga practitioner mastering this art of Tantric Hatha-Yoga.

If you ask people how they would describe the state of happiness and whether or not they see it as a mental or sensual state, the majority of people will classify happiness as a sensual state. If you analyze what is making people unhappy, you will find that an unhappy state is often a result of the disturbances, signals, and sensations coming from the physical body level through hunger, thirst, lethargy, etc. Many of these conditions are making people feel neither satisfied nor happy; the sensations have hijacked the body.

If one learns to control and produce particular body sensations through practicing asanas, vinyasas, and pranayamas organized in special sequences, it is possible to literally build up a physical and energetic balance which brings a true result called inner happiness. Even this experience belongs to the physical state of balance, not a complete conscious state of balance. However, this step is an essential and fundamental part for successful meditation and balancing the fluctuations in the consciousness. It is necessary to pay attention to the sensations of every asana, vinyasa, and pranayama during the practice. It is also essential to learn how these sensations correspond to each other, and how the Universal Yoga® Mandala sequences are balancing the body sensations successfully and bringing the practitioners to a complete conscious state of balance.

All the problems humans have in their lives come from the lack of control over their own consciousness, and one of the main goals of authentic yoga is the development of self-consciousness control. According to the *Yoga Sutras of Patanjali*, an ancient fundamental yoga text, this control of consciousness comes from the ability to stop any mental fluctuations (chitta vrtti nirodha).

That is why it is very important during your practice to accumulate experience to become less mental and more intuitive and sensual. You need to learn to stop the discrimination of the senses and heart by controlling the mind. This is usually impossible during day-to-day life for the majority of modern people.

One of the main meanings of the word "yoga" in Sanskrit is balance. Reaching the balance of a practitioner's physical development, energetic, emotional consciousness, and karmic states is one of the main goals of an authentic yoga practice.

There are different methods in yoga to reach a well-balanced state based on Mantra Yoga (hearing sense), Yantra Yoga (vision sense), and Tantra Yoga (touch sense).

The Universal Yoga® Mandala method joins these three types of yoga together in one practice, increasing the effectiveness of the practice to the maximum possible levels.

The Universal Yoga® Mandala method is designed as a complex series of asanas, vinyasas, pranayams, mantras, and yantras together in one practice. The training sequence is organized as a special mandala structure in multidimensional space.

The integration of the mantras, yantras, and tantras in one mandala practice does not happen immediately, but step by step. In the beginning, practitioners use the mandala sequences including asanas and vinyasas with turns in multidimensional space. Later the sequence incorporates pranayamas, mantras, and yantras, combined with asanas and vinyasas.

Humans have a special organ in their brain responsible for the sense of balance. It is a system of equilibrium. This system registers the human body position in multidimensional space and every turn we make.

For example, if you do a twisting asana during your practice to one side, you will feel a natural imbalance and the wish to repeat this twisting asana to the other side to compensate the feeling of imbalance and return the sense of comfortable balance. Usually practitioners are not doing many twisting asanas during one practice and do not often experience such cases.

It is important for practitioners to make a strong influence at the balancing system by the end of each practice. That is why the Universal Yoga® Mandala method divides the training sequence into sets of asanas, vinyasas, and pranayamas; and during these sets utilizes special turns in multidimensional space to all directions (North, South, East and West).

The sequence represented in this book is not just some random sequence created by me out of well-known asanas and vinyasas. This is a result of decades of practical experiments and perfection of this sequence by me and a group of my best students. The asanas, vinyasas, and pranayamas, as well as all of the turns and general structure of the mandala sequence are precisely chosen. There are a lot of theories and serious methodical reasons for the structure of the sequence represented in this book. It can be the subject of a future book including descriptions of the many important rules of mandala sequencing.

The 4 x 4 Universal Yoga® Mandala Sequence has a short warmup in the beginning. Then there are 16 asymmetrical sets of asanas with turns to different degrees but always to the left on the mat. Immediately following this first series, the sequence repeats the same 16 sets but this time as a mirror reflection by repeating the same asanas but on the opposite side and turning to the right on the mat this time. Every set consists of two asanas. The sets of asanas alternate between leg pairs and arm pairs, then finish with spine pairs.

These 16 sets of asymmetric asanas along with the turns on the mat create a strong sense of energetic imbalance after finishing the first series. The "energetic pendulum" of the practitioner reaches the maximum one side polar point after finishing these 16 sets. It makes a strong influence on the practitioner's system of equilibrium.

The point of developing the strong imbalance at the beginning is to experience the powerful balance at the end. To finalize the practice, there are symmetrical asanas without turns on the mat that increase the sense of balance gained during this well-organized, symmetrical, and balanced mandala sequence.

There are many mandala structures which are possible to build upon to create a sequence. The use of different turning combinations in multidimensional space creates a beautiful geometrical form of yantra for practitioners to visualize. This makes Universal Yoga® Mandala practice an art of Yantra Yoga visualizations.

This particular sequence is a modification of the Static-Dynamic Universal Yoga® sub-style of practice because it uses static stretching and strengthening asanas combined with dynamic strengthening vinyasas during the sequence. It is designed for experienced second level Universal Yoga® practitioners. It can be modified to the more advanced second-third level of Universal Yoga® practice if the practitioner chooses the most advanced variations of the asanas out of those represented in this book. Plus, you have the option of doing a handstand for the vinyasas instead of vinyasa abdomen down or vinyasas side down.

This sequence also develops the quality of physical endurance, based on the high training form, as a result of practicing Universal Yoga® regularly. Practitioners must plan to spend time practicing this sequence. They should avoid running out of energy in the middle or at the end of the practice. Practitioners have to control their energetic state by using conscious breath and making the right exercise intensity choices. They have to develop a state of concentration during their practice, bringing it to the maximum top point at the very end of the practice. Then they have to drop themselves to the deep relaxation state in shavasana at the end of the physical practice. This approach uses the maximum contrast between the active condition and strong concentration during the physical practice compared to the complete passive state and deep relaxation during shavasana at the end of the practice. (After the sequence in this book, shavasana must be between 20-30 minutes.)

Such high contrast of activity brings all energies and the consciousness to a very deep, relaxed, and balanced state.

Then the practitioner sits in a meditation posture with closed eyes to experience "chitta vrtti nirodha" (blank consciousness). When the practice is done correctly, it will be a natural, stable, long, and deep state. (The meditation must be at least 10 minutes, preferably much longer if the practitioner reaches the true stabilization of the consciousness, losing the sense of time.)

When this deep meditation is reached it will make the result of your practice a real yoga practice; accumulating experience of the consciousness control, overcoming the kleshas (roots of sufferings), and reaching all the other important results of the real, authentic form of the Yogic Path.

In the beginning, it is understandable that all practitioners without experience in this particular mandala sequence will practice focused on learning the general techniques of the asanas, vinyasas, and pranayamas. They will be practicing with eyes open or may look in this book for guidance. It is very important to learn all the details of this practice perfectly. Then practice the sequence from memory with eyes closed, without looking at the book even once. This doesn't mean that the practitioner should rush and stop reading the important techniques represented in this book as soon as you remember the sequence itself. It is important to memorize the sequence completely. But it is useful and important also to reread this book a few times, when you are not practicing, to memorize all the important details and techniques of all the exercises and the whole sequence in general.

It can also be useful to read this book again as you continue practicing the Universal Yoga® Mandala Sequence for a couple of months. You will notice that you can understand the information represented in this book on a much deeper level.

When you are able to practice this sequence from memory with your eyes closed, you will remember all of the important techniques represented in this book. Then you will start to build up the state of your consciousness and feel the real wisdom from the teacher's many years of practice, experience, and accumulation of power from this Universal Yoga® Mandala Sequence. You will start to get the real authentic yoga results of the advaita (non-dual) state of your consciousness during each of your practices. You will get the realization of the real meaning of the Yoga Path and the Tantric Method of Mandala Asana Vinyasa practice as a method for your consciousness transformation and development.

All of this experience will be a great preparation for your future Universal Yoga® Internal Practices including mantras, yantras, and the Tantras.

It will change your life. You will be more conscious, leading you to a state of internal happiness. You will be able to use this samadhi (equality) state of your consciousness in the future as a result of your self-control and without having to do any special practices anymore to reach this state. This samadhi state will become the essence of your life. The yoga will be done by you not on the mat only, but at every moment of your life, perfecting the mastership of your existence.

There are seven different samadhi states which can be reached according to the *Yoga Sutras of Patanjali*. Thus the samadhi state which you reach as a result of the Universal Yoga® Mandala Sequence is not the highest samadhi. It will still be samadhi with samskaras (patterns and roots of habits in your subconsciousness). But this will be a samadhi state already, and based on this experience you can perfect it and move to the higher samadhi state without samskaras by practicing the Universal Yoga® Internal Practices in the future.

Here are few additional tips for achieving better results during your practice.

Memorize the sequence so you can follow the Universal Yoga® internal rules of asanas, vinyasas, and pranayamas practice below.

THE RULES OF UNIVERSAL YOGA® PRACTICE:

1. The so-kham or so-ham breath with hushed tone in the throat is always maintained during the practice.

2. The tip of your tongue should always touch the central point of the pallet to the central front point above the top front teeth.

3. Always keep eyes closed during practice.

4. The emotional state and the face must always be neutral and without trying to look nice or to have any other special emotional condition.

5. The attention is always directed to the sensations produced by every asana, vinyasa, and pranayama.

6. Always act out of vairagya; the detachment of the emotions and mind ("the software") from the body and sensations in the body ("the hardware").

7. It is necessary during asana practice to be based on the sensual and not on the mental. Do not think, nor overanalyze, but intuitively understand what is necessary to do to be able to reach the goals of the practice. Act right away on the base of this intuitive understanding of what must be done.

8. All the actions during the practice must to be knowledgeable, effective, and powerful.

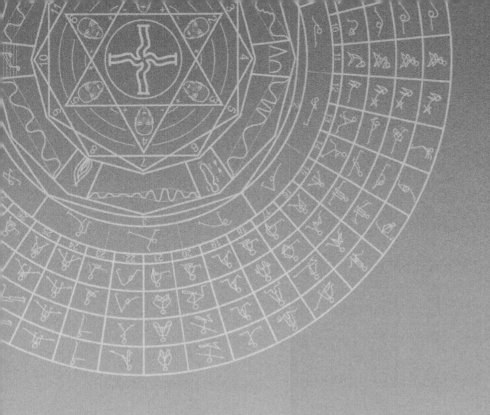

CHAPTER 6

Surrender to the Master

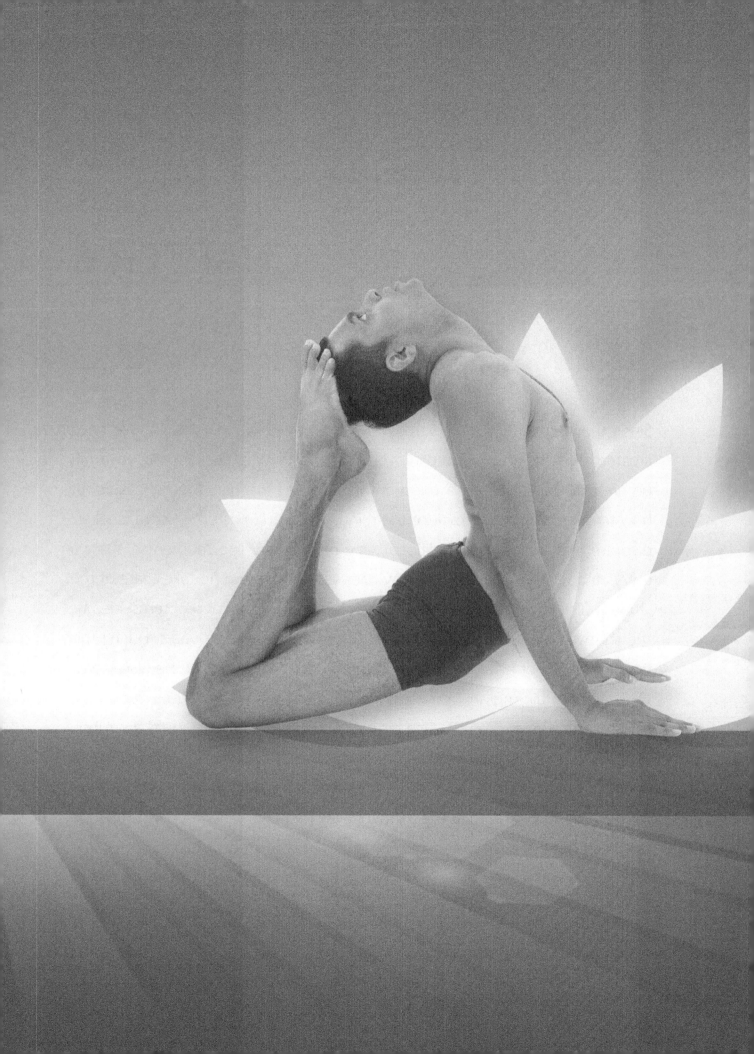

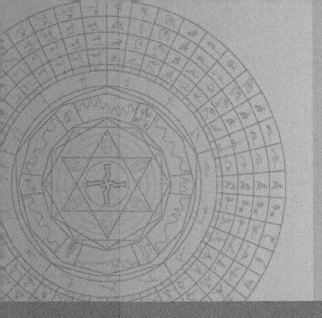

CHAPTER 6

Surrender to the Master

Since the Vedic tradition, India has functioned with a great insight. We have created a system which is used in every form of life. Whatever you do, yoga will be present there. It is not a question of practicing for many hours; it is about how to overcome the turmoil of the mind. The guru (master), shishya (seeker/ disciple) relationship is a traditional way of learning. The moment a shishya enters the gurukul, the responsibility goes to the guru and he takes care of the student. The guru helps the student overcome psychological problems. Ideally, the shishya spends time with his guru for a minimum of 12 years. During this time, he does not just learn postures and breathing techniques. He also learns the way to attain moksha (emancipation). As the shishya develops deep trust towards the guru, he can practice his meditation by using his guru as a symbol. His guru can be his yantra in the same way that he would pray and meditate upon his own desired ishta devata (deity). Focusing the mind towards the guru is tremendous. It helps to fix the mind for a fair period of time. Even an untrained mind can begin this meditation by focusing on his trusted guru. As his trust and practice progresses, he can see the result of clairvoyance and clairaudience in a very short period of time. The power of guru does not lie in the guru. It lies in the disciple. He attains success not because of the power of his guru, but because of the power of his strong trust.

The main concept is we have a guru who has reached the ultimate essence; in other words, he has reached a suprarational experience. Through that experience he, or she, is able to guide people in the right direction. He is a mystic, a sage, a yogi! A guru is one who is not interested in the outer world. On the contrary, he consciously drops the outer world. Though his concern is not about being in the outer world, still he is able to travel through it without any distraction. In India, we follow this lineage everywhere, independent of whichever ashram you join. That is when a disciple receives initiation (diksha) from a guru. If the disciple is such that he has an interest to grow on the internal level, he must be able to have shraddha (complete trust) towards his guru. The guru will not cling to you forever, nor will you be under the guru's guidance forever. It is just a matter of time. Once the disciple matures or ripens, it is possible that the guru will send the disciple away to share his experience around the world.

Such lineages have continued from the Vedic period up until now. However, the bond between the master and disciple is an inexplicable experience. It functions from the state of love, but not from the state of control. For these reasons, in the East we don't have a high suicide rate. The reason behind that is because if we have any mental or emotional issues, we don't go to a hospital. Instead we go to a guru where the problems can be resolved, and the family can go back home happily.

The guru plays a major role in the field of yoga and liberation. Now, in the modern world, yoga is possible for everyone. This is a fair and great opportunity for everyone. On the other hand, nowhere do you see internal peace. Today, teaching yoga has simply become another sort of corporate job. Although some wonderful teachers are maintaining the lineages and striving towards the path of enlightenment, the majority of yoga instructors are proposing only physical postures without having any idea about the student's physical and mental condition. In such cases, yoga has merely become physical instruction rather than the path through which one strives to be a master over both the body and the mind.

A guru will rekindle your inner potential regardless of your weakness. He meticulously helps his disciple transcend the intellectual mind into experiential patterns that lead the disciple to overcome all sufferings and anxieties. The guru's presence is extraordinary. Basically, he is an alchemist. He can turn copper into gold. That is how it is in the East in all the ashrams. We have satsang (a spiritual discourse). Satsang is one of the important parts which can be played by the role of a teacher. In satsang, the guru can simply shatter the disciple's ego. It is like he can shed some light into the darkness.

That is another meaning of the word "guru" as well. The guru is one who removes all darkness. It is the biggest operation the guru performs on his disciple. This operation does not happen out of control or with aggression. It happens out of pure love and compassion. Once the job is done, and if the disciple is ready and matured, he not only leaves his master, but also carries on the lineage. He shares and transmits his knowledge to others as well.

Guru:

An Alchemist.

For a Western audience, praising a guru this much is shocking. In the West, some may have their idol, teacher, or mentor. But in the West, there is a concept of equanimity. Teaching is about treating everyone equally. Equanimity is the way.

In the East, when a student studies under a guru, he first encounters some painful memories. A teacher will test you in all circumstances to ensure that your visit to the ashram is to learn and realize the Self. A guru will take you out of your comfort zone and lifestyle. In my childhood, when I was learning with my guru, he tested me for many months to ensure that I was really invested heart and soul in learning. The teacher wanted to confirm that my learning was neither by parental force nor just for fun.

The guru tests your sincerity during your learning period. Based on that, he will or will not impart his knowledge to a disciple. In modern yoga studios, we can see many times that the student controls the teacher. In return, the teacher has to comfort the student so as not to lose the student. Because a student can walk out and learn in another place, the teacher could possibly lose a student and their income as well. Therefore, such teachers comfort the student's ego by always being overly nice to them. It is sheer hypocrisy. It leads nowhere but to the state of schizophrenia. A self-realized guru will not create this drama. He would rather whack you and give you a hard time to ensure that you are out of your comfort zone. The guru will not pamper the student ego. On the other hand, regardless of how strict the guru is, you are still enchanted by his actions, and he will pull your attention just like a piece of iron is attracted and pulled toward a magnet. A guru functions like a mother. It is not his ego that seeks to destroy your ego. Rather it is his heart's desire for you to shine like a light. It is no different than a mother who restrains a child's bad habits. A child can go astray in so many ways. A loving mother is strict with her child when the child is about to fall into the pits and traps of life. Just because she is strict with the child doesn't mean she doesn't love him/her. On the contrary, it is tough love that a mother uses to protect her child from falling into any pit. Similarly, being strict with students doesn't mean that the teacher is trying to control the students. The teacher is protecting the students from the darkness in the unconscious realm of the mind. He guides the student to find their own inner source. Please understand it's not about making a war with the mind, as the mind is not the enemy. Rather, the enemy is some unconscious clutter clinging its way into our conscious mind. We are trying to change that pattern through understanding, not fighting.

Because of societal relationships and the education system, we are constantly bombarded by many moral rules and ethics. For example, the people whom you want to be upset with will simply not allow you to be upset. Rather, they will teach you to smile despite being upset. You are not forced to follow this strategy, but it becomes our daily life process. We become accustomed to such unconscious, hypocritical actions and we think that they are real! But suddenly a guru comes and wakes you up from the long years of such unconscious sleep. That is why it is hard to change the old pattern of the mind, even though the mind knows it's a good change. Our daily habits still tether us here. We live literally like a plastic flower, and here comes the guru telling us how to live like a real rose rather than a plastic one. You must learn to enjoy the fragrance of the rose he creates as a steady position in you. He will guide you to organize your own body and mind connection.

This lesson is important to everyone. Students needs a guru to pull them back to center. This is real maturity. Such maturity will lead you to find your own inner guru. When you can find your own inner guide, you are freed from your outer guru. Even if you want to be with your guru, he will not allow you to be with him anymore. The outside bond might be broken, but the guru has given his flesh, blood, and soul to his student. The heart-to-heart communion is alive. That is how the parampara (guru-shishya tradition) has been kept alive until now.

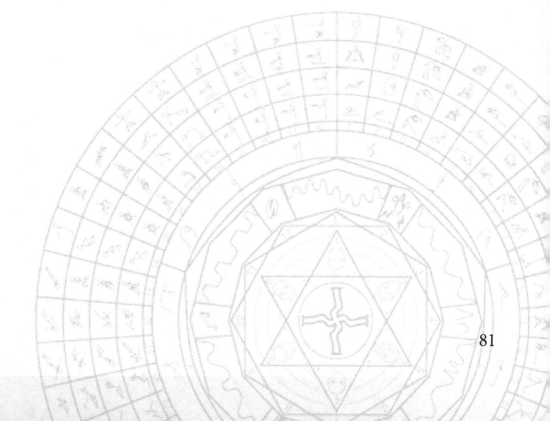

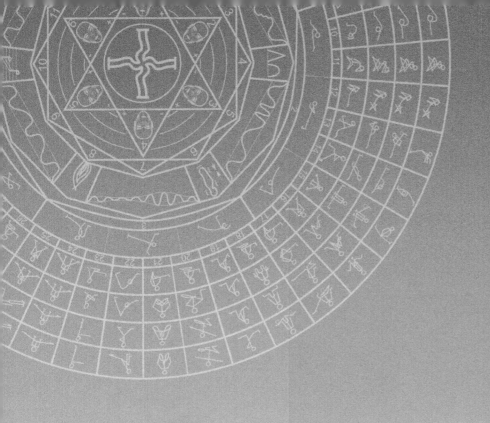

CHAPTER 7

Asana and Vinyasa

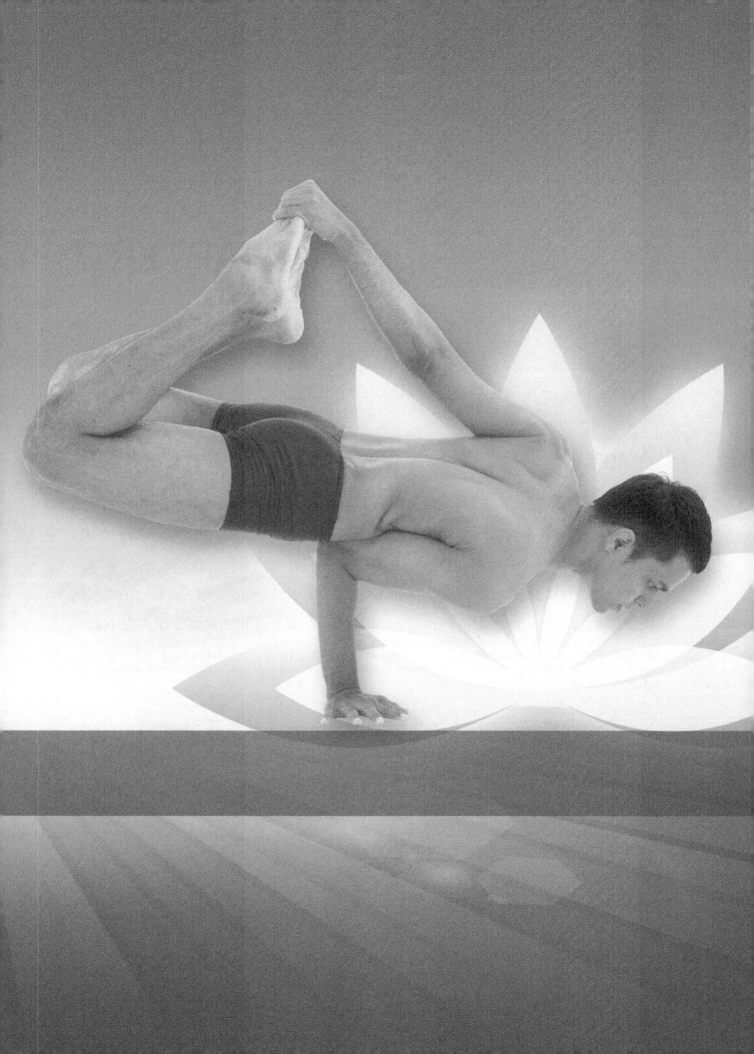

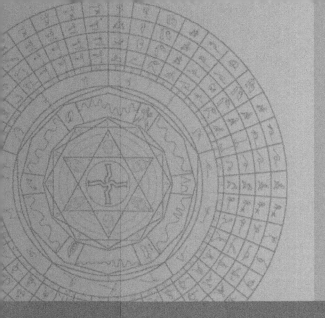

CHAPTER 7

Asana and Vinyasa

The Journey of Asanas from the Ancient Tradition to the Modern Tradition

Asana:

According to Patanjali, the word asana means seated pose, an undistracted posture while you are sitting. Even before Patanjali, there were texts explaining asanas that mainly focused on meditative purposes, which they referred to as a seated posture. In the primitive state of practice, asana was done by sitting long or dangling on the branches of the trees. In ancient traditions asana existed for example in Hinduism, Jainism, and Buddhism.

In *Yoga Chudamani Upanishad*, asana is mentioned as the first step. In the *Gheranda Samhita* asana is mentioned as the second step among seven steps. According to the *Hatha Yoga Pradipika*, "Asana is the first state of liberation from the cycle of rebirth." In Thirumoolar's *Tirumantiram,* asana is listed as eight seated positions such as sukhasana, svastikasana, padmasana, simhasana, sthirasana, virasana, bhadrasna, and siddhasana. *Gheranda Samhita* mentions about 32 asanas. Some traditional schools mention as many as 86 asanas. In Nepal and Tibet, there are many asanas ingrained in the temples and monasteries. In Delhi, there was a popular teacher called Dhirendra Brahmachari who describes 108 asanas. In 1984 B.K.S Iyengar, who was a student of Tirumalai Krishnamacharya, published his famous book, *Light on Yoga*, which includes more than 200 asanas. And in 2003, Dharma Mittra himself managed to publish a poster with 608 postures, which later was made into a book.

Asanas are continuously evolving. Although some lineages work with many asanas, other schools use very few. In their teaching of yoga, some schools emphasize the sun salutation, which is a sequence of asanas that link one position to another. They can be practiced separately and also combined with gazing methods which we call drishti. Fixing the mind in asana is one of the most important goals of yoga.

Asanas can be perfected gracefully, helping to regain your health, and improve your body's range of motion. Many students have practiced asanas (postures) as a first path of yoga; that's how the modern studios propose yoga. Distinguishing stretching from strengthening can guide you and keep your practice in symmetry. Regular practice with repetition is essential, and that's the only way to adapt your asanas quickly. With regular discipline, effort starts reducing along with the physical tension created in the beginning. Consequently, you begin to understand the physical aspect of your body and become conscious of your body's movements. Furthermore, as you progress you can even isolate, strengthen, and stretch specific muscles consciously.

"Without a perfectly healthy body one cannot gain bliss."

-Hevajra Tantra

Here we emphasize that the body needs to be fit and healthy to attain the higher state of consciousness. A weak body simply cannot sit and have a deep state during internal practices. By practicing asana and pranayama, you are preparing your body as a vehicle to fly higher. Your practice is such that, in the beginning you have to put in effort, and through that effort it is possible to reach the state of effortless practice. In the beginning the body reacts with discomfort, which is good. But if you stop progressing the next day just because it hurts, then your growth can never reach any height.

This is why regular practice is necessary; it simply takes your weakness away. Once your body gets used to the asanas, vinyasas, and breathing techniques, you will feel lighter and start responding to your practice. For this experience, one needs an experienced teacher who has the proper education and has mastered the asanas him/herself. Only then is it good to propose the practice to a student. An inexperienced instructor may injure the student because he doesn't know how the pose can fit into the body, and wrong moves can put the student at risk. Therefore, analyze your teachers carefully before you commit yourself to them for your own practice.

- For one who masters it, your body and mind are no longer the source of pain and distraction. Only after you are in absolute harmony with yourself is it possible to prepare for the higher spiritual sadhanas.
- In this sequence, we aim to attain a balanced state of practice that helps to work on your whole body, breath, mind, and spirit.

Vinyasa:

Vinyasa means movement, a link between the external movement of the body and internal movement of the breath combined with the invisible part of our mind. One can experience movement through non-movement, or in Taoism they call it "an action through inaction." In all religions there are some form of movements which are intended to create the coordination for our body, mind, and spirit. We begin to understand that in the name of physical practice, we have a form of expression that brings us closer to reality.

Vinyasa is a moving meditation, just like the Dance of Shiva®, modern dance, karate, wrestling, samurai, archery, or running, etc. Similarly, vinyasa can create a steady unwavering flow of awareness. The goal of vinyasa is not to master the movement but to be absorbed and become one with the movement. On this planet everything is moving. The whole universe is created out of movement. Just like planets orbit the sun and electrons spin around the nucleus, so the heart is constantly pulsating around 60–70 gallons of blood throughout the body. It is pumped out and travels around the body and returns back to the heart in 23 seconds. Breath is constantly moving in and out, and the mind is in a constant flow of thoughts. Everything is flowing; therefore, dynamic movement-based techniques are not something that yogis have discovered carelessly.

It's a conscious technique produced by human intelligence. Yogis have discovered these methods for every type of personality. Before one can practice, he or she must be able to know his/her individual mindset. If your mind is running aimlessly and never willing to sit and focus for a fixed period of time, then begin your practice with vinyasa, which is a dynamic form of yoga. As your movement helps you fix your mind, you will become focused by the end of your practice. When you become dedicated in movement, you are able to see the whirlpool of the mind gradually becoming steady and fixed. You can initiate your dynamic meditation method with some visualization methods. This will give you a taste but don't stop there. Bring your awareness into all your activities. It's like you are opening the curtain of a window, and as you open it you can see the ray of sunlight passing through your window. The concept is the same here. When you bring more light into your practice and into your daily activities, your quality of life will improve and will not be the same as it used to be!

In Tibetan Buddhism, movement-based visualization is very important. In order to master the mind, one must be able to understand the movement of the mind and engage the mind through movements itself. Through movement, one can transform his way of life. In my teacher Andrey Lappa's book, *Yoga: Tradition of Unification*, he talks at length about the vinyasa system and different styles as well as creative, eloquently-designed vinyasas. In this century it has been the only book that explains vinyasa in a very detailed way.

Common attributes to ignite the catalyst in you.

Time to practice:

The best time to practice is early in the morning. You can begin with Shiva Nata® (Dance of Shiva®) to start your sequence. (Shiva Nata® is described in great detail in Andrey's book *Yoga: Tradition of Unification*). In India, we had to wake up at 4 am to start our sadhana (spiritual discipline) and finish it before 7 am. If you don't have time in the morning, then at least practice in the evening, which will lead you to progressive growth and success.

Wear loose clothes:

Wear any loose clothes that can make you feel that the cloth is not a barrier for your practice; avoid wearing tight or uncomfortable clothes.

Dietary Rules:

In the morning, drink a glass of room temperature or lukewarm water with lemon. Strictly avoid cold water. Before you begin your sequence, ensure your bowels are evacuated and your bladder emptied. While you are practicing, you are awakening your fire energy, therefore, don't stop the energy that you have created by drinking water. Strictly no diet sodas or any soft drinks. If you are practicing in the evening, a three to four hour gap after lunch is necessary. Strictly avoid practicing right after your meal as the acid reflex will invade your esophagus and can eventually cause heart burn, bloating, burping, or even nausea, which in turn can lead to dyspepsia or chronic stomach disorder.

Right Environment:

It is always important to practice in a calm and quiet environment. Choose a place where you can separate yourself from your family and avoid internet connections. Isolate yourself from all gadgets, friends, and families. Either practice in an empty room or in a studio where you have freedom to practice. Avoid direct sunlight and avoid practicing in a cold room; no air conditioner is required while you are practicing.

Self-practice comes with a greater discipline as it can add immense value to your spiritual sadhana. In the beginning of your learning period, it is good to practice under the right guru who can lead you to better understand your alignments, as well as rejuvenate your perceptions from a guru's vision. This is one attribute which the East has immensely. Right now we have an overload of information available in the media. It takes away the possibility of learning from the right guru or the possibility of being the right student. Now the media promotes more on the marketing success; you can see a lot of teachers who call themselves gurus on the Internet. This increases the risk of students just acquiring information versus learning to explore deeply the changes that can happen within. The guru's presence will enhance the vibration and reverberates in each and every cell of your body, whereas learning through online classes only will not do justice to the whole potential and allow a seeker to grow in all attributes. Therefore, learning directly from an experienced master is needed in your search. This search is very important for an aspirant; only then will you go in the right direction towards your goal. Once you know what your goal is then you can develop in that aspect by maintaining your practice on a regular basis. Self-practice will improve your asana practice, which is tailored to your physical needs.

Benefits of Self-practice:

- Build up your regular physical practice, which cultivates confidence based on self-discipline.
- Improves your decision-making skills.
- Enhance your practice by working on your weaker zones. Whether it is asana, pranayama, or even internal practices, it eventually leads you to enhance and establish your quality of practice substantially.
- Explores new research to work on your body in a better way.
- You can adjust the time of practice which brings freedom in choosing a practice time.

Hindrances of Self-practice:

- Avoid being overly competitive as you could end up having injuries, but nevertheless every injury is a lesson to be learned.
- For a beginner who is learning, avoid comparison between you and other senior students as it can make you feel inferior towards your practice.

- If you have any existing injuries or difficulties you are encountering, then allow the simplified version of the postures to be adapted rather than hard movements.
- You could have the best environment, but if your frame of mind is not right then your practice could drift away. If you are feeling lazy it's easy to skip practice, instead do your regular practice to create discipline in your body and mind.

Overcome Injury:

Pain is inevitable during asana practices. It varies from pose to pose. Some people might be flexible by nature, whereas some might be flexible doing forward bends, but not so flexible in backbends, etc. The best possible way to avoid injury is to know your body well and listen to your body. Body memory is very strong, and each time you do your practice, find the areas of weakness and strength in your body. Severe strain can cause muscle, ligament, or tendon injury. Sometimes the accumulation of emotions can cause damage to the body as well. It is important to find out the causes of the issue. Whether it is a small or big injury, be more connected towards the body and listen to the body's response. During asana practice when the body is not ready but the mind wants to do the pose because others are doing it, be mindful to avoid severe injury and depression. While you are on the mat doing some poses, know well that when the muscles indicate certain pain is unbearable or causing sharp pain, that's the signal the body gives you to stop your movements from pushing harder. The sequence that you have here and the asana photos that you see in this book may not be the same when you practice the postures. It can vary depending on your body proportion, age, experience, and how often you practice. Based on this, your practice varies.

This book is not given to copy the exact pose that I am doing here. One day you might feel flexible, whereas another day you may feel stiff. Just analyze your practice and learn according to your body's condition. Not all poses are necessary for one to do here; rather it's the body's capacity that it can go beyond its limit as well. You can get injuries from over adjustments by your teacher, or you can injure yourself by pushing harder. In both cases the victim is you. If the injury was inevitable then at least avoid your practice for a period of time until the damage has been repaired. If it is a long term injury, seek medical advice or physical therapy. In this case don't stop your practice totally; on the contrary, strengthen the weaker muscles. It is better to start your yoga practices sooner than later. While you are in the middle of the practice and the body feels tired and needs rest, it's better to rest the body. There is no need to enforce your asana practice so intensely when the body is not ready at all. Rather, go through other aspects of the practice. A long pranayama practice or long dhyana practice can compensate your regular sadhana. Give some time to your body to adapt and adjust, then you can better enjoy this sequence with minimum risk of injury. Remember yoga is the key to drop all your sufferings; the first suffering to avoid is weakness and illness in the body.

From the outside shavasana looks like the easiest technique ever, but when you are into the position you will learn how hard it is to be still and relaxed. Shavasana is one of the important ancient techniques in yoga. If any muscles are tensed and tight, it can impede your relaxation. If the breath is erratic, shavasana helps to bring your breath back in control as your belly starts moving in and out. Shavasana can bring greater results by reducing stress, lowering blood pressure, and keeping the senses calm. But remember, it's not a state that leads you to sleep. You are in a resting position yet totally awake and aware of your surroundings, not concentrating on anything in particular, a state of non-doing, which is why it works best right after your physical practice.

Time of practice:

If you are practicing this sequence for 3 hours, then be aware that your relaxation time should be at least 20 to 30 minutes. Here you are not simply lying down with some thoughts overflowing. The aim of this practice is to break the habit of old thought patterns. Therefore, during shavasana, allow deep relaxation by shutting down your sensory perceptions, not allowing them to function the way your mind might want to. Allow your sensory perceptions to settle down so that you can reintegrate your body and mind together.

Avoid intense and strenuous practices during menstruation and pregnancy. It may also be important to avoid inversion postures. Always seek advice from a medical professional for contraindications. If you have limitations, ask your teacher to modify this sequence as needed.

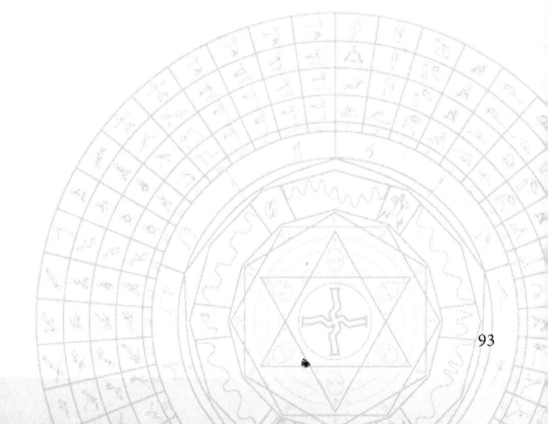

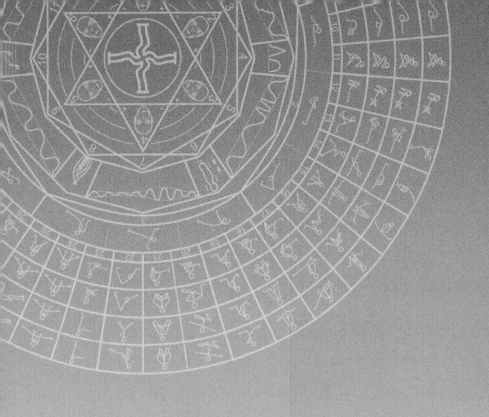

CHAPTER 8

4 x 4 Universal Yoga® Mandala Sequence

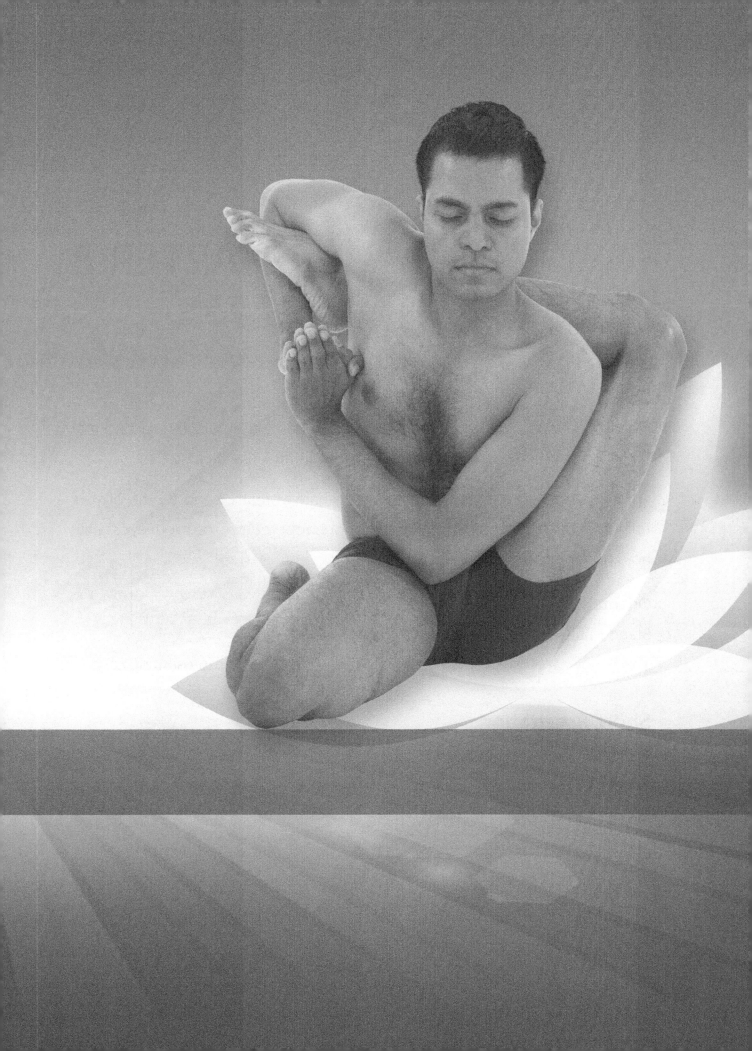

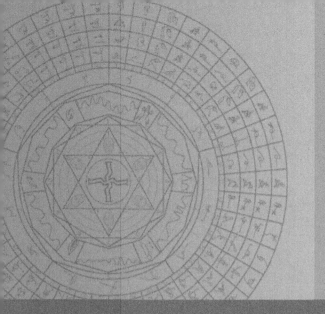

CHAPTER 8

4 x 4 Universal Yoga® Mandala Sequence

Note:

Place one mat on the floor in the transversal plane, then place a second mat on top in the longitudinal plane. Your mats will look like a cross.

Throughout practice maintain a steady "so-ham" breath. Keep the tip of your tongue to the roof of your mouth behind your front teeth. Close your eyes while holding the poses.

Orientation:

Stand in the center of your mat facing forward.

This is now what is considered the direction on your mat representing East.

Short Prostration:

Surrender to the universe.

Stand in tadasana, keep your feet together, arms at your side. Inhale and raise your arms over your head and bring your palms together (Figure: 290). Exhale and lower down placing your knees, palms, and forehead on the floor (Figure: 291). Stretch your arms out to prostrate to the universe and your teacher (Figure: 292). This is a gesture of complete surrender to the universe and to your ego-maker. To return, bend your elbows. Inhale, lift your head, stand up and bring your arms overhead, palms together. Exhale and bring your palms together at the center of your chest (Figure: 293).

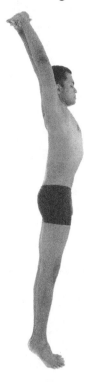

Figure: 1

Tadasana:

Tad: palm tree

How to enter:

From short prostration, stand up keeping your feet together. Interlace your fingers, turn your palm upwards, raise your arms overhead, and as you inhale, elongate your whole body. Lift your heels up and balance on the balls of your feet (Figure: 1). Fix your attention on one point or close your eyes and gaze inward. Hold and balance for six breaths.

* Start of Beginning Set:

You will be repeating this set on the other side.

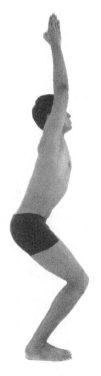

Figure: 2

Utkatasana:

Utkata: fierce, proud. Also called chair pose.

How to enter:

Stand with your feet together. As you inhale, bend your knees and lower your hips in a relaxed state, as if you are sitting on an imaginary chair. Keep the back of your spine long and avoiding arching the lower back. Stretch your arms up and press your palms together with your elbow straight. Tilt your tailbone forward slightly and bend your knees further without straining (Figure: 2). This is one of the dynamic methods of pushing the inner energy towards an upward direction; therefore, maintain for eight to twelve long breaths.

Ardha Chakrasana:

Ardha: half; chakra: wheel, it resembles half wheel position, hence the name.

How to enter:

Stand with your feet apart, place your palms on the side of the lower back. Inhale and lengthen the spine up; as you exhale, gently lift the chest and arch your spine in a backward motion. Keep the legs straight and slightly engage your belly muscles without straining (Figure: 3). Hold for six breaths and release.

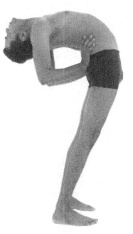

Figure: 3

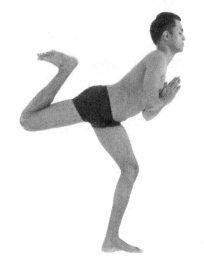

Figure: 4

Kavadiasana:

Kavi: saffron; adi: foot. Another meaning behind this is that the devotee carries a large wooden decorated arch around his shoulders from his home to the temple, or from one temple to another temple, resembling a symbol of purity or an act to destroy one's own ego.

How to enter:

Stand on your feet equally, bend your torso forward slightly with your hands in prayer position at the middle of your chest. As you inhale, lift your right leg behind you, flex your knee and foot, keep your hamstrings engaged, and bring your heel closer to the buttocks. Keep the left knee slightly bent and arch your spine. Keep your chest lifted and push the back foot up higher (Figure: 4). Maintain balance between the torso and leg. You can close your eyes and hold steady once you have mastered the pose. Stay for six breaths and release.

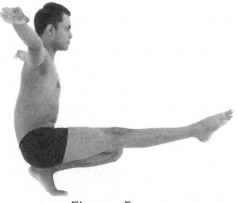

Figure: 5

Eka Pada Vakrasana:

Eka: one; pada: foot; vakra: bent

How to enter:

From kavadiasana, move your right leg forward, keep it straight, and place your left sit bone on your left heel. Maintain an upright position of your torso and extend your arms back, placing the fingers in jnana mudra (Figure: 5). Take six deep breaths. If you find it hard to balance without support, place your fingers on the floor to the sides of your body and hold steady.

Ardha Chandrasana:

Ardha: half; chandra; moon. This pose represents a half moon.

How to enter:

Stand with your feet together, arms overhead. Catch your left wrist with your right hand, left fingers in mushti mudra (thumb is placed inside the edge of the pinky

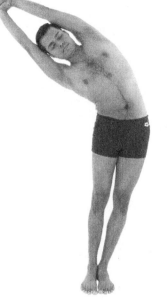

Figure: 6

finger and close the other fingers). Inhale and lengthen the spine up. As you exhale, bend your body to the right. Keep your chest lifting up, pelvis in a neutral position, and legs straight. Pull the left arm to the right keeping the neck neutral. Keep your nose facing forward (Figure: 6). Fix your gaze at one point or close your eyes. Stay for six long breaths. This ends the first side of the beginning set.

* Mirror Reflect the Beginning Set:

Repeat the five poses (Figures: 2, 3, 4, 5, and 6) now on the opposite side then continue on to ukatasana.

Utkatasana:

Stand with your feet together equally and repeat the directions as it was previously explained (Figure: 2).

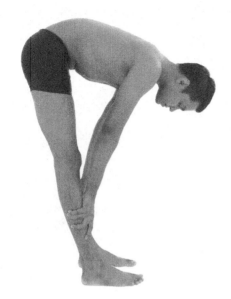

Figure: 7

Uttanasana:

Ut: intense, deliberate; tan: stretch, lengthen.

How to enter:

Variation 1:

If your back is stiff or your hamstrings are tight, then use this simple option. Keep your hands on your ankles and bend your torso forward. Keep your chin back. Don't force the spine to lengthen. Stay for a few breaths.

Variation 2:

Padahasthasana:

Pada: foot; hasta: hands. In this pose your hands will be placed under your feet.

Stand with your feet hip distance apart. Elongate your spine as you fold your belly toward your thighs. While exhaling, bend forward and place your palms under the bottom of your feet. Stand completely on the palms and lean forward slightly, press the feet firm, and pull the arms to the side of your body. Now move your head towards your knee caps, keep your abdomen firm but not in a tensed state, and do not strain the neck. Stay for six to eight long and steady breaths.

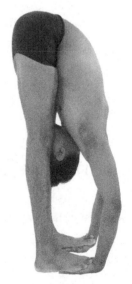

Figure: 8

Vinyasa:

Vinyasa Abdominal Down:

From padahastasana, inhale the head up, place your palms on the floor, and exhale while jumping back into a plank position. Then follow the next steps.

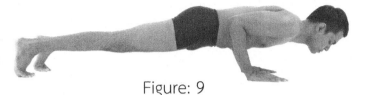

Figure: 9

Step 1:

Chaturanga Dandasana:

Chatur: four; anga: limb; danda: a staff

From plank position, bend your elbows and lower down into a low plank position called chaturanga dandasana (Figure: 9).

Step 2:

Urdhva Mukha Svanasana:

Urdhava: upward; mukha: face; svana: dog

Here you enter this pose from chaturanga dandasana. As you inhale, raise the body up, keep the shoulders straight, and lengthen the spine to arch the back. Slightly push your chest forward and look up without collapsing your neck. Keep your legs engaged and avoid holding your breath (Figure: 10).

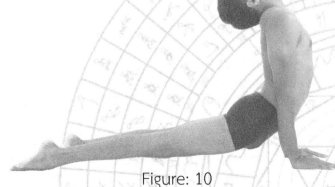

Figure: 10

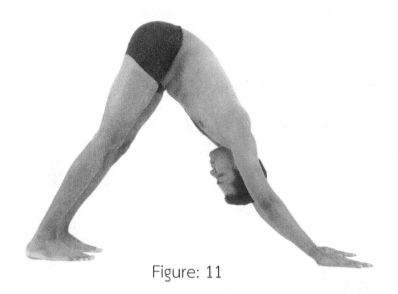

Figure: 11

Step 3:

Adho Mukha Svanasana:

Adho: downward; mukha: face, svana: dog

From urdhva mukha svanasana you are directly entering into adho mukha svanasana. Your feet are hip width apart and your hands shoulder width apart. As you exhale press your feet on the floor and move your head toward your feet, stretching your arms. Avoid rounding your lower back, relax your belly muscles, and keep the neck in a neutral position without tension. Gently turn your thighs in and press your heels firmly on the ground (Figure: 11).

Turn:

From adho mukha svanasana (Figure: 11) jump legs wide and turn left 90 degrees.

Orientation:

Face the direction on the mat representing North.

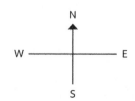

Asanas:

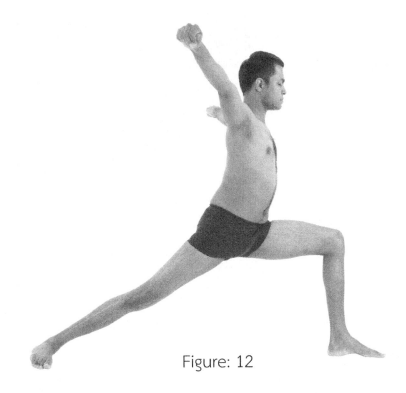

Figure: 12

Virabhadrasana:

Virabhadra: warrior (a heroic warrior)

How to enter:

From adho mukha svanasana, step your left leg forward as you inhale. Then bend your left knee 90 degrees. Turn your right foot inside from a 90 degree to 45 degree angle and press the foot down firmly on the floor, but be careful not to put extra pressure on the right side of the knee. Keep the torso up firm and gently turn your chest to face forward. Expand your arms to the sides and as if you are pulling your arms backwards. Place your hands in mushti mudra. Avoid tensing your shoulders, and withdraw the shoulder blades down. Keep your hips squared by pushing your right hip gently forward. Close your eyes and gaze inward for the next six long breaths.

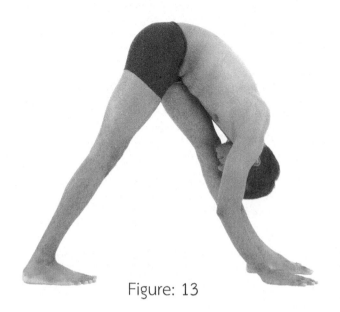

Figure: 13

Trikonasana:

Tri: three; kona: angle. This is the Universal Yoga® version of triangle pose.

How to enter:

From virabhadrasana, bring your back foot half a step forward and push the back heel down, keeping both feet pointing forward. As you exhale, bend forward, lengthening the spine and neck. Place the left shoulder in line with the left shin bone. Keep both feet firmly grounded on the floor. Place your palms on the floor with your fingers in line of your left toes. Avoid stretching the arms forward. Hips should be neutral in this pose. Close your eyes and gaze inward for the next six long breaths.

Note:

If your hamstrings are stiff, then put your hands on your shin or ankle and rest in the pose.

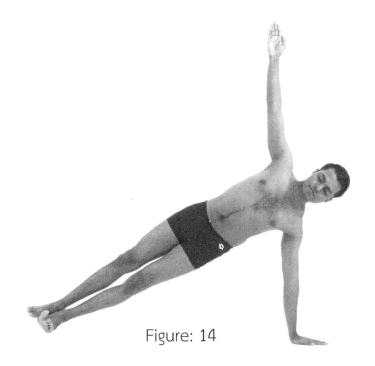

Figure: 14

Vinyasa:

Vinyasa Left Side Down:

From trikonasana, step back to plank position and lean on your left hand and prepare for vinyasa left side down.

Step 1:

Inhale and turn your body to face sideways. Your left arm is on the floor and right arm is up in the air, head and nose directing straight forward. Place your right foot on top of your left foot (Figure: 14). If your arm is not strong enough to support you yet, step your right foot forward and place it on the floor in front of you to provide support.

Step 2:

As you exhale, lower your left hip toward the floor without resting on the floor and simultaneously move your right arm down with your elbow bent, keeping your palm facing up (Figure: 15).

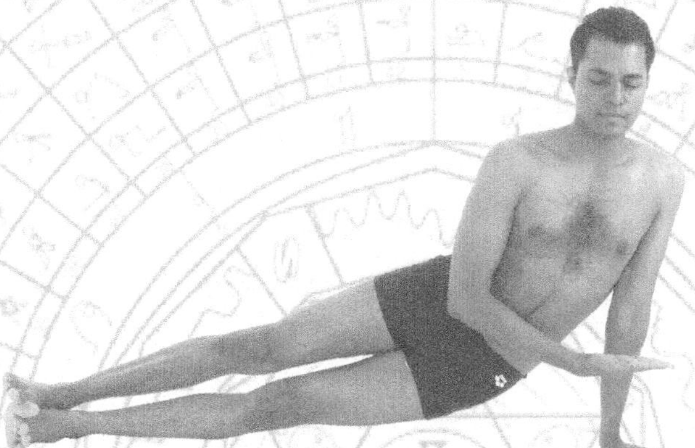

Figure: 15

105

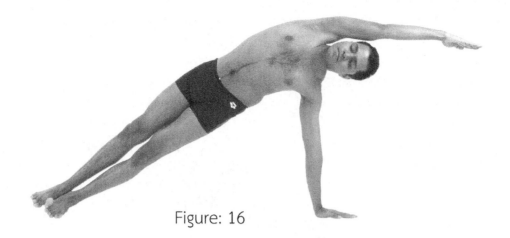

Figure: 16

Step 3:

As you inhale, lift your hips high and stretch your right arm over your head. Legs are straight and sharp in position (Figure: 16).

This completes one round. Do one round each time you do this vinyasa.

Turn:

From vinyasa left side down, bring your right leg forward placing your right foot next to your left hand, which is holding the weight of your body, press the right foot into the floor and turn to the left 180 degrees.

Orientation:

Face the direction on the mat representing South.

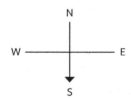

106

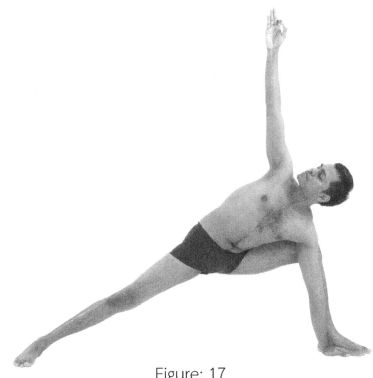

Figure: 17

Asanas:

Utthita Parsvakonasana:

Utthita: lifted or extended; parsva: side; kona: angle. Extended side angle pose.

How to enter:

Inhale and bend your left knee, keeping the quadriceps engaged. Your left knee should not go beyond the line of your left ankle. Bring the left palm to the floor inside your left foot. Allow space for your ribcage so you can breathe with ease. Draw your shoulder blades down your back towards the hips.

As you lengthen the spine in a diagonal line, stretch your right arm up and keep the right hand in jnana mudra. Turn your head up to gaze at your right fingers. Don't let your thigh sink down. Stretch your right leg back spinning the outside of your heel down. Press your feet firmly into the floor. Keep both legs firm and maintain balance between the work of the left and right legs. Close your eyes and gaze inward for six long and soft breaths.

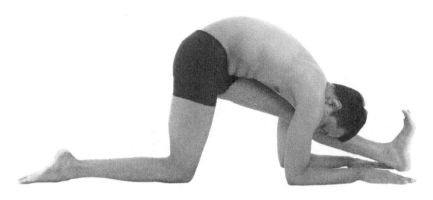

Figure: 18

Ardha Trikonasana:

Ardha: half; tri: three; kona: angle

How to enter:

From utthita parsvakonasana, enter into ardha trikonasana by lowering the right knee down and stretching the left leg out straight. As you exhale, fold forward towards your left shin bone. Keep the right thigh vertical maintaining a 90 degree angle at the knee (Figure: 18). Draw the belly in slightly. Avoid rotating your left thigh outward, instead keep it rotating inward a little to keep toes pointing straight up. Bend forward until you can place both elbows on the floor evenly. Flex your left foot to access the maximum stretch for your leg. This is the beginning state to prepare your body for more advanced poses. The right pressure will allow you to improve the range of flexibility on your hamstrings, but avoid straining. Stay for six long breaths. Keep your eyes closed and gaze inward.

Note:

If your hamstrings are tight. Stay on your hands rather than trying to bring the elbows to the floor. Listen to your body and gradually allow the body to increase its range of flexibility through regular practice.

Vinyasa:

Vinyasa Left Side Down:

From ardha trikonasana, (Figure: 18) step back to plank position and lean on your left hand and prepare for vinyasa left side down.

Now repeat vinyasa left side down one time (Figures: 14, 15, and 16).

Turn:

From vinyasa left side down, bring your right leg forward placing your right foot next to your left hand, which is holding the weight of your body, press the right foot into the floor and turn to the left 90 degrees.

Orientation:

Face the direction on the mat representing East.

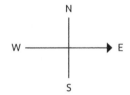

Asanas:

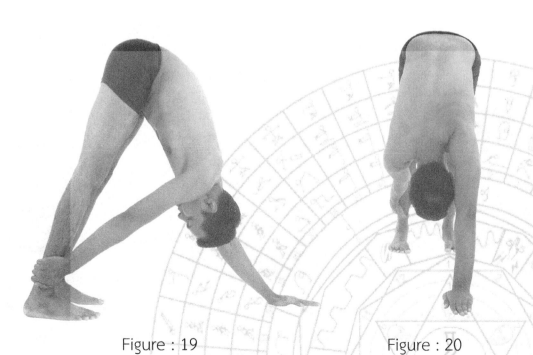

Figure : 19   Figure : 20

Eka Bhuja Adho Mukha Svanasana:

Eka: one; bhuja: arm; adho: downward; mukha: face; svana: dog

How to enter:

From adho mukha svanasana, keep your feet hip distance apart and bring both feet one step forward. Keep your pelvic girdle neutral while lengthening your spine as much as you can. Keep your quadriceps engaged. Grab your left ankle with your left hand. Gently press your right shoulder backwards simultaneously pushing the left shoulder forward (Figures: 19 and 20). This keeps your shoulders in a neutral position. Activate the shoulder girdle, outer deltoids and forearms. Avoid hyperextension of your right elbow. Hold for six breaths.

Eka Bhuja Nidanikasana:

Eka: one; bhuja: arm; nidanika: rack.

From eka bhuja adho mukha svanasana (Figure: 20) turn left 180 degrees, lifting your left leg up a few inches and spin your left leg above your right leg allowing you to sit on the floor with feet flat. You are now facing the direction representing West. Enter into eka bhuja nidhanikasana.

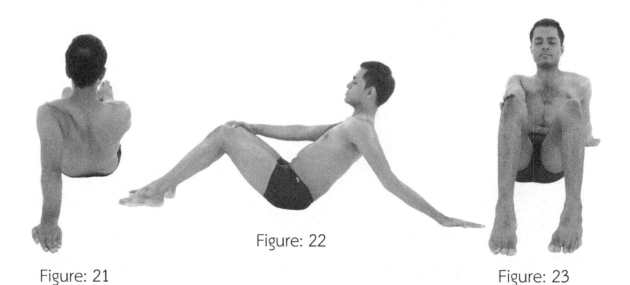

Figure: 22

Figure: 21

Figure: 23

How to enter:

Variation 1:

After completing the 180 degree turn and sitting on the floor your right fingers are facing away from your feet. Place your left hand on top of the left thigh and lengthen your spine. Now gently push your right shoulder forward and pull your left shoulder backward to bring your shoulders in a neutral position (Figures: 21, 22, and 23). Avoid slipping on the right side of your arm, hold your right hand firmly on the floor. This pose stretches the front of the shoulder. It strengthens and firms the trapezius and shoulder girdle region.

Stay for six long breaths. Then turn right 180 degrees coming back to the starting point in eka bhuja adho mukha svanansna.

Variation 2:

This is an advance variation of the same pose.

After you master the first variation place your left elbow on the floor and lift the spine up. Keep the head in the central plane of the spine (Figures: 24 and 25).

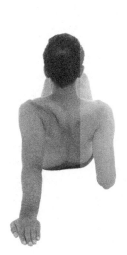

Figure: 24

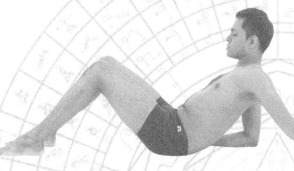

Figure: 25

Vinyasa:

Vinyasa Left Side Down:

From eka bhuja adho mukha svanansana (Figure: 20), step back to plank position and lean on your left hand and prepare for vinyasa left side down.

Now repeat vinyasa left side down one time (Figures: 14, 15, and 16).

Turn:

From vinyasa left side down, bring your right leg forward placing your right foot next to your left hand, which is holding the weight of your body, press the right foot into the floor and turn to the left 180 degrees.

Orientation:

Face the direction on the mat representing West.

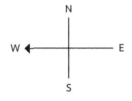

Asanas:

Eka Bhuja Swastikasana 1:

Eka: one; bhuja: arm, swastika: an ancient symbol which resembles good fortune and represents the four seasons.

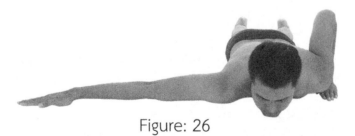

Figure: 26

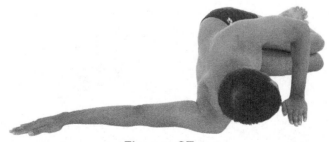

Figure: 27

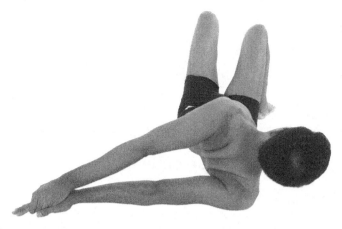

Figure: 28

How to enter:

Variation 1:

Lay on your stomach and stretch your right arm to the side, with the hand as high as the crown of your head. Keep the palm facing down and avoid placing the hand over the head (Figure: 26). Gently lean onto your right hip leaving the right shoulder rotating externally. Pull the knees gently in towards the line of your hips. Place the left palm on the floor, elbow bent up to the ceiling (Figure: 27).

As you externally rotate your shoulders more freely, then lift both knees up and place your buttock on the floor, standing on the soles of your feet. Now gently bring your left arm behind your back and grab your right forefingers with your left hand. Push your legs towards the hands using the legs as a leverage to stretch the right shoulder more deep and effectively (Figure: 28). In the beginning it might be hard to grab your fingers, particularly if you have a stiff shoulder or other shoulder issues. Therefore, play with it carefully and avoid over stretching the shoulders.

Note:

If this pose is accessible then you can prepare for the advance movements using the same side. Choose any one position and hold for six long breaths. Advance variations are only done if you have experience doing this sequence regularly.

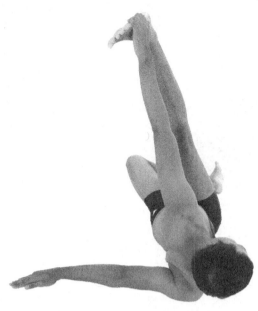

Figure: 29

Advance Variation 2:

This is a deep external rotation stretch of the shoulder. Lift your right leg up and grab your outer edge of your foot with the support of your left hand (Figure: 29) moving the left knee down towards your right hand. Allow the right foot to move towards the line of your right hand.

Advance Variation 3:

Grab your right forefingers with your left hand and gently press your left elbow on top of your right elbow (Figure: 30) to encounter a deep stretch.

This is an incredible stretch for the pectoralis muscles, front deltoids, and side of the torso.

Note:

If you have suffered a shoulder injury such as rotator cuff or labrum tear, consult your personal yoga teacher for further assistance.

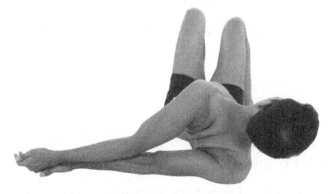

Figure: 30

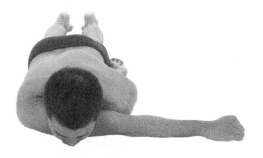

Figure : 31

Eka Bhuja Swastikasana 2:

From eka bhuja swastikasana 1 (FIgure: 28), lay on your stomach and keep the legs together, head in line with your spine. Avoid leaning on the side.

How to enter:

Variation 1:

As you exhale bring your right arm under the throat, rotating the right shoulder internally and keeping your right elbow straight. Now bring your left arm next to the right thigh (Figure: 31) and press your left shoulder down towards the right arm. Avoid choking the throat. Rest both hands on the floor, in mushti mudra, right hand facing down and left hand facing up.

Variation 2:

From eka bhuja swastikasana 2 (Figure: 31), move your right leg out to the line of the hip and press the left shoulder further down towards the right arm, or place your right shoulder on the floor (figure 32). Place your chin on the central plane of your spine. This helps to stretch your deltoids, latissimus dorsi, trapezius, and forearm together.

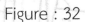

Figure : 32

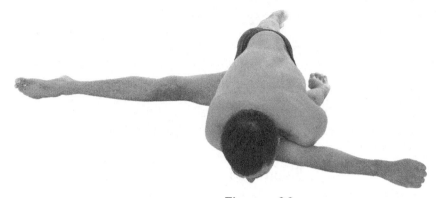

Figure: 33

Variation 3:

Keep the right leg back and as you exhale flex your left hip, crossing your left leg below your right leg. Rest the left outside of your thigh on the floor in a horizontal position towards the right side (Figure: 33). Press your right shoulders down on the floor and don't raise the shoulder joints up. Then place your left anterior shoulder on top of the left arm, keeping your hands in mushti mudra with your right wrist facing down and left wrist facing up. Stay for six long breaths.

Variation 4 :

This is a deep internal rotation of the shoulder. Bring your left leg under your right leg from below and lay on your left outer hip. Your right arm is stretched under the throat. Bend your left knee keeping the outer region of the hip resting on the floor. Place your right ankle in front of your left thigh, bringing your

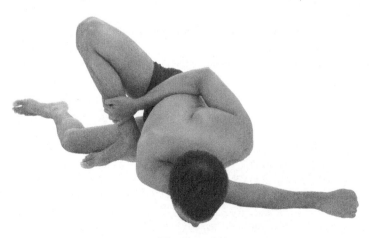

Figure: 34

right foot onto the floor, moving into half lotus position (Figure: 34). You need to have a deep thoracic twist of the spine. Avoid holding your breath. Now bring your left arm behind your back and grab your right shin bone.

Variation: 5

Follow the same steps as mentioned for variation four (Figure: 34) except change the legs into full lotus position on your left side (Figure: 35). Start by bringing your left leg on top of your right thigh. Then place your right leg on top of your left thigh resting your right foot on the floor. Now grab your left foot with your left hand, placing your left shoulder on your right forearm.

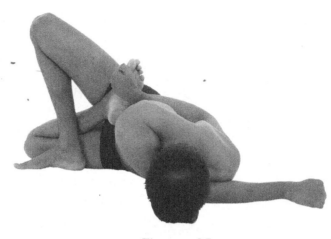

Figure: 35

Note:

In order to master these advanced variations (Figures: 33, 34, and 35), your range of mobility for the shoulders, pectoralis minor, latissimus dorsi, and external obliques should be quite flexible. Avoid the temptation of doing this position without further warmups or without prior experiences.

Vinyasa:

Vinyasa Left Side Down:

From eka bhuja swastikasana 2 (Figure: 31) step back to plank position and lean on your left hand and prepare for vinyasa left side down.

Now repeat vinyasa left side down one time (Figures: 14, 15, and 16).

Turn:

From vinyasa left side down, bring your right leg forward placing your right foot next to your left hand, which is holding the weight of your body, press the right foot into the floor and turn to the left 180 degrees.

Orientation:

Face the direction on the mat representing East.

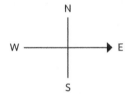

Asanas:

Ashwa Sanchalanasana:

Ashva: horse; sanchalana: stepping movement. Also called equestrian pose or runner's pose.

How to enter:

As you exhale, bend your left knee keeping it in line with your left ankle and

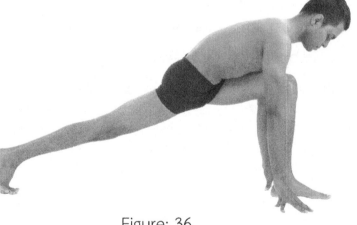

Figure: 36

place your fingers on the floor. Firm your right thigh and knee to keep the back leg straight and balance on the ball of your right foot (Figure: 36). Lengthen your spine. Stay in the pose for six long breaths.

Hanumanansa:

A powerful devotee of Rama; also called the monkey god

How to enter:

Variation 1:

From runner's pose enter into hanumanasana by moving your left leg further forward stretching your hamstrings. Push your right pelvis forward to create a neutral line of your hips. Flex your left foot and extend your right leg backward (Figure: 37). One must have a deep external and internal rotation of the hips. Don't let the back leg slack. Bring awareness to both legs which will give you a sense of grip in the pose with less effort.

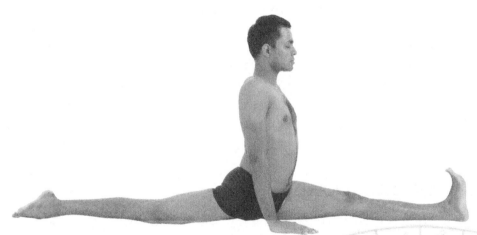

Figure: 37

Variation 2:

Bend forward and catch your left heel with your hands. Don't lean to the side (Figure: 38). Maintain balance and distribute your weight evenly.

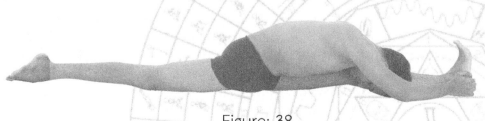

Figure: 38

Variation 3:

If you are able to do hanumanasana easily, then grab your left ankle with your right hand and bring your left arm under the throat, keeping the left hand in mushti mudra, with palm facing down. Place your forehead on your right forearm, keep the left arm straight and simultaneously gain more access towards your hamstrings and buttocks. (Figure: 39). Now stay for six to eight deep breaths.

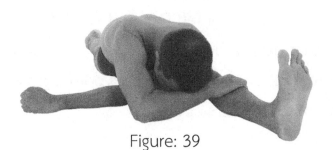

Figure: 39

Vinyasa:

Vinyasa Left Side Down:

Exit hanumansana (Figure: 38), step back to plank position and lean on your left hand and prepare for vinyasa left side down.

Now repeat vinyasa left side down one time (Figures: 14, 15, and 16).

Turn:

Bring your right leg forward and turn to the left 180 degrees.

Orientation:

Face the direction on the mat representing West.

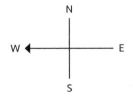

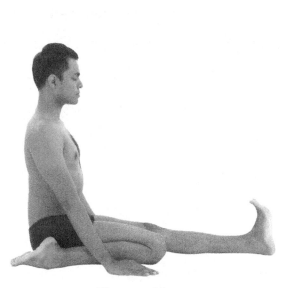

Figure: 40

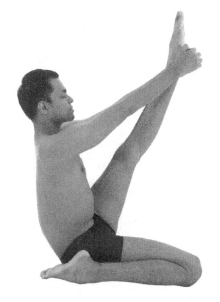

Figure: 41

Asanas:

For this asana you can choose from a variation of krounchasana or viranchasana.

Krounchasana (Option 1):

Krouncha: heron.

How to enter:

Variation 1:

Lower your right knee to the floor and sit to the inside of your right ankle, while pulling your right calf out of the way. Your toes will be pointing back, in ardha virasana (half hero pose). Keep the left leg straight (Figure: 40). Bend forward, grab your left leg, and lift it up (Figure: 41). Pull your left shinbone towards the left shoulder. Keep your foot in plantar flexion (Figure: 42).

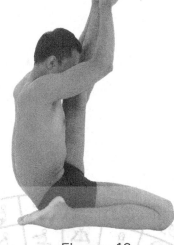

Figure: 42

Variation 2:

Apply the same principles as it was shown in (Figures: 42 and 43). Then grab the left outer edge of your foot with your right hand and place your left palm on the floor with the fingers facing front. Pull the left leg behind the left shoulder

121

and lengthen your back and neck (Figures: 43 and 44). Avoid lifting the left sit bone up keeping your hip into neutral position. Stay for six breaths.

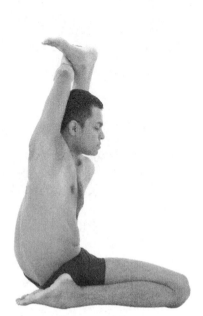

Figure: 43

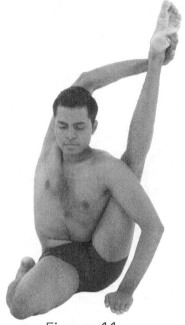

Figure: 44

Viranchasana 1 and 2 (Option 2):

Resembles the name of the brahma.

How to enter:

To do viranchasana 1 you need to have good external rotation of your hips, strength in your neck, and good shoulder mobility.

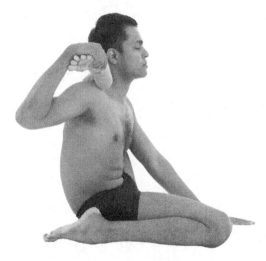

Figure: 45

Variation 1:

Bend your right knee and sit on the floor, with your right toes pointing backwards in plantar flexion. As a result, your right leg will be in virasana position. Grab your left ankle with your right hand and bring your left leg back behind the shoulder. Bend your left knee and catch your left ankle with both hands to get a deep external rotation of your left hip. Now slightly bend the torso to bring the left leg behind the neck. Use the back of your shoulders to nudge the left lower extremity of the leg downward towards the scapula, simultaneously keeping the back and neck active (Figure: 45). Avoid rapid breathing, instead keep it slow and steady. While you keep the left foot pointing forward in plantar flexion, bring your hands in namaste mudra (Figure: 46). This pose involves deep internal rotation at the right hip and deep external rotation

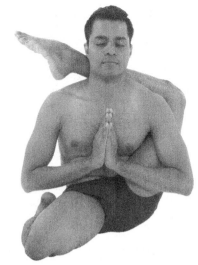

Figure: 46

at the left hip joint. If you are trying to master the advance version of bringing your right arm over your left leg, you must be able to do virasana without any effort. Check if you feel pressure on your knees. If you do, then do not practice the advance steps without guidance from an experienced teacher.

Variation 2:

Follow the previous steps for viranchasana (Figure: 45). After the left leg comes behind the neck, extend your right arm up and bind it on the left foot joining your hands in namaste mudra on the lateral side of your chest. (Figure: 47 and 48). Stay for six breaths.

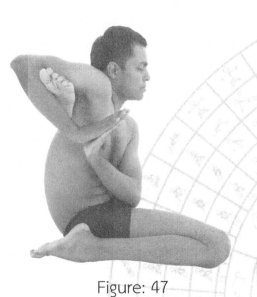

Figure: 47

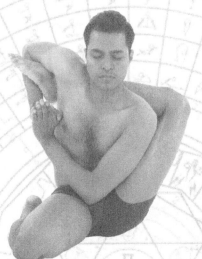

Figure: 48

123

Ardha Padmasana:

Ardha: half; padma: lotus.

For ardha padmasana, you can practice all of the variations from the previous pose, adding the same steps as explained for krounchasana or viranchasana.

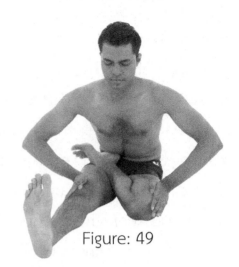

Figure: 49

How to enter:

Variation 1:

From a seated position with straight legs, bend your right knee and place your foot on top of the left edge of your upper thigh. Once you place your leg in half lotus pose, then gently squeeze your legs in (Figure: 49). Don't push too strong on your knees. Now fold your torso forward, catch the heel of your left foot with your hands. Rest your right shoulder on top of your right knee. Rest your head on the floor (Figure: 50).

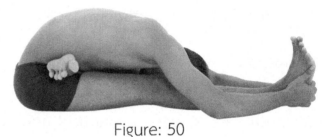

Figure: 50

Variation 2:

Ardha Baddha Padmasana:

Ardha: half; baddha: bound; padma: lotus.

Follow the same principles mentioned in the previous variation. Then bend your left elbow and bring your left arm behind your back to grab your left foot. Fold forward catching your right heel with your right hand Figure: 51). When you

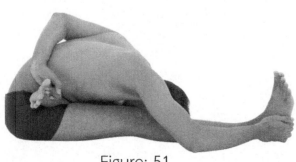

Figure: 51

are ready to add on, lift your leg up (Figure: 52). Pull your left shinbone towards the left shoulder. Keep your foot in plantar flexion and lengthen your spine. Stretch your hamstring deeply.

Variation 3:
Ardha Padma Eka Pada Sirsasana:

Ardha: half; padma: lotus; eka: one: pada: foot: sirsa: head.

Follow the same principles mentioned for viranchasana 1 (Figure: 46) except have your right leg in half lotus position.

Variation 4:
Ardha Padma Eka Pada Kapilasana:

Ardha: half; padma: lotus; eka: one: pada: foot: Kapila: Vedic sage.

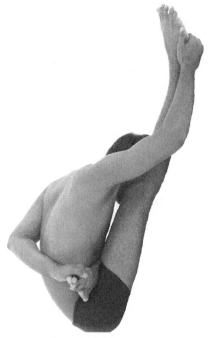

Figure: 52

Follow the same principles mentioned for viranchasana 2 (Figure: 48) except have your right leg in half lotus position.

Vinyasa:

Vinyasa Left Side Down:

Release from ardha padmasana and bring the right leg back into ardha virasana so you can lunge forward. Then step back to plank position and lean on your left hand and prepare for vinyasa left side down.

Now repeat vinyasa left side down one time (Figures: 14, 15, and 16).

Turn:

From vinyasa left side down, bring your right leg forward placing your right foot next to your left hand, which is holding the weight of your body, press the right foot into the floor and turn to the left 90 degrees.

Orientation:

Face the direction on the mat representing South.

Asanas:

Eka Bhuja Padmasana

Eka: one; bhuja: arm; padma: lotus.

Here you are going to do the practice lotus position with the support of your arms, hence the name of the pose.

How to enter:

Step 1:

Lay on your stomach and keep your legs together. Your head should be in line with your spine. Avoid leaning to one side.

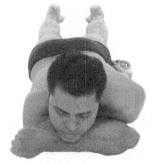

Figure: 53

Step 2:

As you exhale, cross your right arm under the throat directing it to the left placing the arm in line with the shoulder (Figure: 31). Bend your right elbow bringing the extensor side of the wrist (ulnar bone), which is the line of the pinky finger, under your central part of the chin. Don't choke your throat by placing the wrist under the throat (Figure: 53). Bring your left arm next to the left thigh, resting it on the floor. Press your left shoulder down towards the right forearm. Keep both hands in mushti mudra. Your left palm should face up whereas your right palm should face your shoulder.

Step 3:

Sweep your right leg forward in line with the hip. Press the right shoulder further down towards the left forearm or

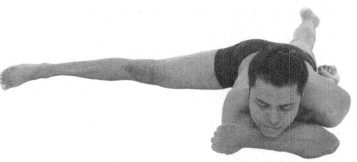

Figure: 54

place your right shoulder on the floor (Figure: 54). Keep your chin in the central plane of your spine. This can help to stretch your anterior deltoids, pectoralis minor, latissimus dorsi, trapezius and forearm. Stay in the pose for six breaths.

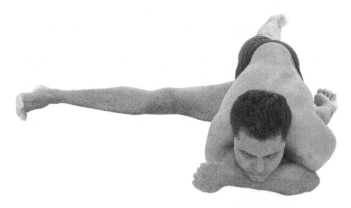

Figure: 55

Advance variation 1:

Take a deep exhalation, then flex your left hip and cross your left leg underneath the right leg. Your left outer thigh should rest on the floor in a horizontal position. Keep your right leg straight back (Figure: 55). Press your right shoulder down onto the floor. Avoid lifting the shoulder joints up. Rest your left anterior shoulder on top of the right forearm. Rest your left hand on the floor. Keep both hands in mushti mudra. Your left palm should face up whereas your right palm should face your shoulder. Stay for six long breaths.

Advance Variation 2:

This position creates a deep external rotation of the shoulder joint. Take a deep exhalation, then flex your left hip and cross your left leg underneath the right leg. Your left outer thigh should rest on the floor in a horizontal position. Keep your right leg straight back. Slide your right arm under your throat, then bend your right elbow keeping your right wrist under the chin in lotus of the arm position. Keep your right hand in mushti mudra. Now bend your left knee 90 degrees. Then go into half lotus position by placing your right ankle in front of your left thigh bringing your right foot on the floor (Figure: 55). This creates a deep thoracic twist of

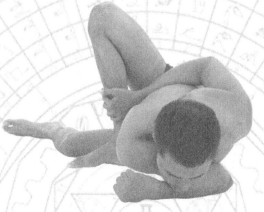

Figure: 56

the spine. Avoid holding your breath. Now bring your left arm behind your back and grab your right shinbone. If this position puts too much pressure on your shoulder, stop the advance methods or seek guidance from an experienced Universal Yoga® teacher.

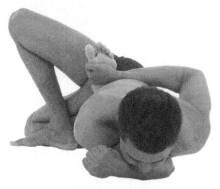

Figure: 57

Advance variation 3:

Follow the steps as mentioned in the advance variation 2 (Figure: 56). Here change the legs into full lotus position on your left side. First bring your left leg on top of your right thigh and place your right leg on top of your left thigh, resting your right foot on the floor. Now grab your left foot with your left hand, placing your left shoulder on your right forearm.

Note:

To master these variations, you must have good range of mobility in the shoulders. Plus, the pectorals minor, lattisimus dorsi, and external obliques should be quite flexible. Avoid the temptation of doing this position without mastering the first variation. Regular practice can bring you into a state of effortlessness, calmness, and ease.

Eka Bhuja Virasana:

Eka: one; bhuja: arm; virasana: hero. Virasana pose is typically done in a sitting position to activate the hips and legs, which includes the knees and ankles. In Universal Yoga®, the same concept is used to activate the shoulders and arms, including the elbows and wrists. This represents hero in the form of arms.

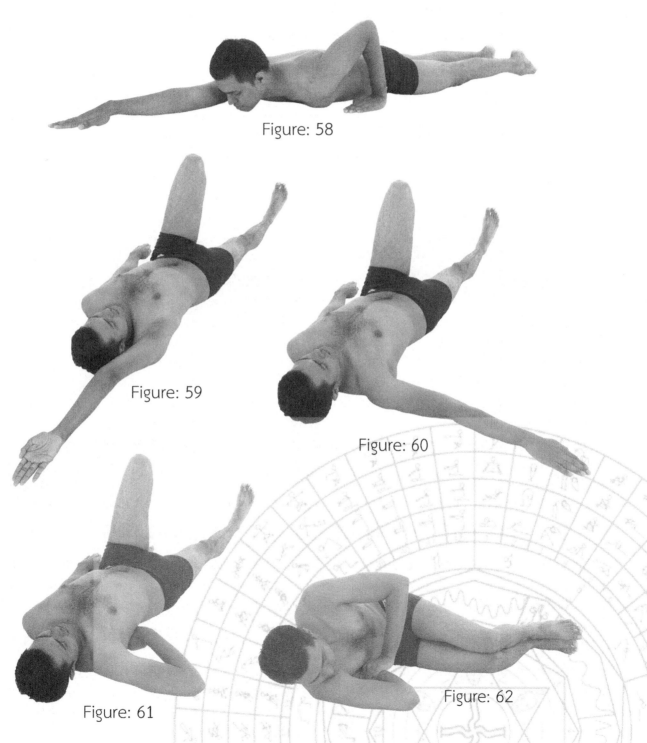

Figure: 58

Figure: 59

Figure: 60

Figure: 61

Figure: 62

How to enter:

Exit from eka bhuja padmasana and once again lay on your stomach. Direct your right arm over the head (Figure: 58). As you inhale, roll over on your buttocks keeping the left knee bent (Figure: 59). Now bring your right arm to the right side in line with your shoulder (Figure: 60). Keep the right palm facing down, flex your elbow, and place your right palm under the right armpit (Figure: 61). Here you get a fair amount of medial rotation of your right shoulder. In order to go deeper into this pose, exhale and roll onto your right outer hip and thigh, pull both knees towards your hips, press your left palm on top of your right wrist bone, and avoid raising the right shoulder up. Keep the right outer shoulder on the floor (Figure: 62). Stay for six breaths.

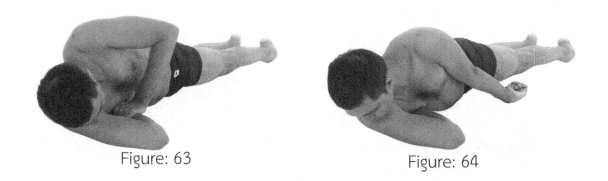

Figure: 63   Figure: 64

Advance variation:

Follow the steps from the previous variation until you've placed your right palm under the armpit and rolled over onto your belly, but keep both legs straight (Figure: 63). Then keep your left arm straight, pushing your left shoulder slightly down towards the line of your right elbow. Your abdomen will come in contact with the floor. Keep your left wrist facing up in musthi mudra (Figure: 64). Avoid holding your breath.

If you are an advance practitioner, then try this pose but do not hurt your joints. This pose gives you a deep internal stretch on your posterior deltoid, teres major, subscapularis, and supraspinatus.

Vinyasa:

Vinyasa Left Side Down:

From eka bhuja virasana, step back to plank position and lean on your left hand and prepare for vinyasa left side down.

Now repeat vinyasa left side down one time (Figures: 14, 15, and 16).

Turn:

From vinyasa left side down, bring your right leg forward placing your right foot next to your left hand, which is holding the weight of your body, press the right foot into the floor and turn to the left 180 degrees.

Orientation:

Face the direction on the mat representing North.

Asanas:

Eka Bhuja Kapotasana:

Eka: one; bhuja: arm; kapota: pigeon. Pigeon pose is typically done with the legs, knee bent 90 degrees with a rotation of the hip. In Universal Yoga®, the same concept is used to activate the shoulder. This represents pigeon in the form of arms.

How to enter:

Step 1:

Lie on your stomach, keep both legs straight, bend your right elbow, and bring it to the right side of your waist. Keep

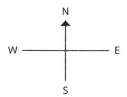

Figure: 65

131

your right elbow on the floor with the palm facing down. Now direct your left arm straight in line with your left shoulder, placing your left palm down (Figure: 65).

Step 2:

Bend your left elbow halfway so your left forearm is vertical. Press the left palm down, fingers pointing to the left (Figure: 66).

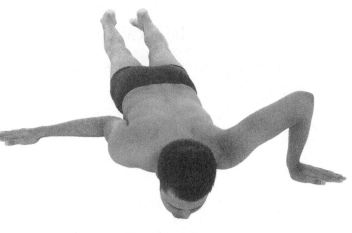

Figure: 66

Step 3:

Bend your right knee and place your knee on top of your right forearm. Keep your left leg straight. Use the left arm as a lever to lift your left shoulder up simultaneously pressing your right shoulder down. Your chin should face down on the floor in the central plane of the spine (Figure: 67).

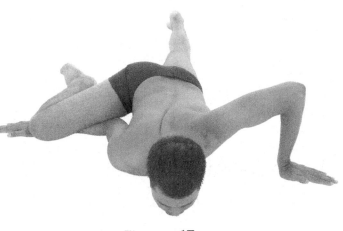

Figure: 67

This is a lateral rotation of your right shoulder, which is an incredible practice to stretch your infraspinatus, teres minor, and pectoralis minor.

Advance variation:

This advance asana should only be practiced by someone with good range of mobility in both shoulders. Start by bringing both knees onto the forearms, and press your chin down on the floor (Figure: 68). Avoid turning your head as it can reduce the level of the stretch and can create imbalance.

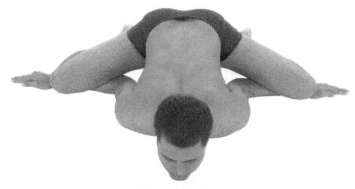

Figure: 68

Eka Bhujasana:

Eka: one; bhuja: arm.

This pose helps improve the stretch of your right elbow and forearm.

How to enter:

Step 1:

After you exit from eka bhuja kapotasana bring both legs together in a squat. Keep your feet hip width apart. Turn your right palm to face backwards so your fingers face you. Place your right knee on top of your right upper arm.

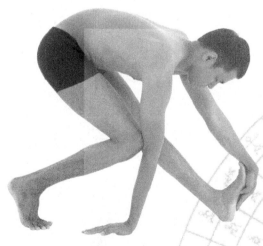

Figure: 69

Step 2:

Now stretch your left leg out and grab the ball of your left foot with your left hand. Pull your left leg back and press your right knee forward. In the beginning it is fine to rest your right sit bone on top of your right heel. If that is accessible, raise your hips high and slightly pull the right elbow back to avoid extreme hyperextension on your right elbow (Figure: 69). Hold for six breaths.

Vinyasa:

Vinyasa Left Side Down:

From eka bhujasana, step back to plank position and lean on your left hand and prepare for vinyasa left side down.

Now repeat vinyasa left side down one time (Figures: 14, 15, and 16).

Turn:

From vinyasa left side down, bring your right leg forward placing your right foot next to your left hand, which is holding the weight of your body, press the right foot into the floor and turn to the left 180 degrees.

Orientation:

Face the direction on the mat representing South.

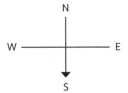

Asanas:

Eka Pada Kapotasana:

Eka: one; pada: foot; kapota: pigeon. One legged pigeon pose is a modified version of full pigeon pose. Here the emphasis is on the lateral rotation of your left hip.

How to enter:

Variation 1:

Lower down to the floor and flex your left knee to 45 degrees (Figure: 70). Place hands firmly on the floor and keep your hips level. Stretch your right

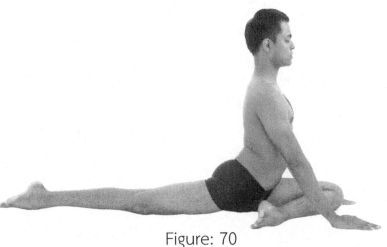

Figure: 70

leg back keeping the knee pointing down and while elongating your spine.

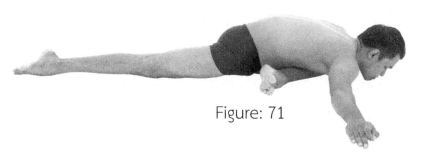

Figure: 71

Then, fold your torso forward moving your arms out to the sides in line with your shoulders. Place your palms down with your hands in jnana mudra (Figure: 71). Avoid leaning to the side of your left hip. Keep your torso symmetrical by applying equal pressure on both hands and keep the back leg straight. If you have tight hips, this is a good way to start working on your hip flexibility.

If you encounter lateral cruciate ligament issues then place a block under the left sit bone or seek an experienced Universal Yoga® teacher for guidance.

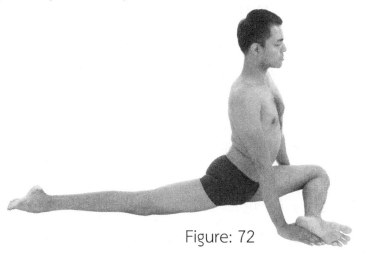

Figure: 72

Variation 2:

Apply the same principles as in variation 1 with a slight change. Simply bend the left knee further forward from a 45 degree to a 90 degree angle. Maintain the dorsiflexion of your left foot; this can protect the lateral side of your knee joint (Figure: 72). Make sure the knee is free from any pain, then gently bend forward keeping your arms out to the sides.

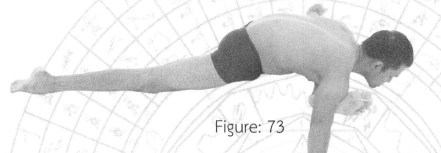

Figure: 73

Avoid lifting your left buttock up and press your right leg firmly on the ground. Lengthen your spine, keeping your chin on the central plane of your spine (Figure: 73). In the beginning stay for a minute or two. Once you get familiar with this posture, hold for six breaths.

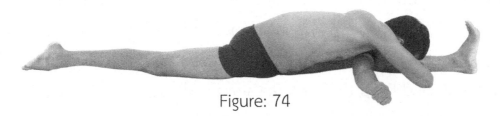

Figure: 74

Hanumanansa:

This pose is dedicated to sage Hanuman, also called the monkey god.

How to enter:

Step 1:

Now enter into hanumanasana by spreading your left leg further forward to stretch your hamstrings. Push your right pelvis forward to create a neutral line of your hips, flex your left foot to point the toes up, and extend your right leg pointing your toes back (Figure: 74). You need to have deep external and internal rotation at the hips. Don't slack the back leg, bring awareness to both legs.

Step 2:

Fold forward catching your left heel with your hands. Maintain balance and distribute your weight equally, avoid leaning to the side. If you are able to do hanumanasana well, then grab your left shin or ankle with your right hand and bring your left arm straight under your throat keeping your left hand in mushti mudra with the palm facing down. Place your forehead on your right

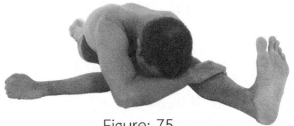

Figure: 75

136

forearm simultaneously gaining more access in your hamstrings and buttocks (Figure: 75).

Advance variation 1:

From hanumanasana, flex your back knee catching your foot with your right hand. Then spin your right hand and fingers to face forward in the same direction as the right toes, placing your palm on the top of your right foot. Keeping the right foot in plantar flexion, use the pressure of your hand to press your right foot under your waist. Then grab the left ball of your foot with your left hand, raise your chest high, and keep your neck in line with the rest of the spine (Figure: 76). Once you have your balance, gently push your right hip forward to avoid leaning to the left side.

Advance variation 2:

This advance variation creates a deeper asymmetrical stretch of the legs. You must have flexible hamstrings and the ability to flex your knees deeply through diligent practice.

To start, apply the same principles as shown in advance variation 1. Then, medially rotate your right leg to hook your right foot under your 12th right rib or waist effortlessly. Do not lean to your left. Now either place your hands on the

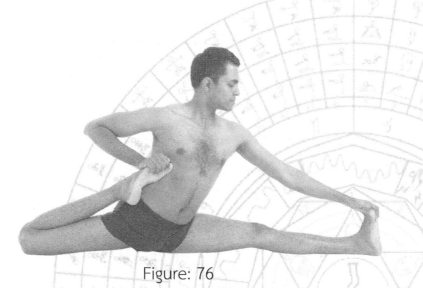

Figure: 76

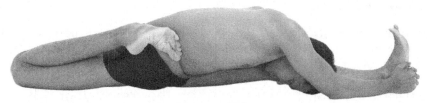

Figure: 77

floor trying to balance, or lean forward and catch your left heel by resting your elbows on the floor (Figure: 77). Stay for six breaths.

Then, gently release the right foot from your waist, sweep your left leg back, go into high plank pose to prepare for the next vinyasa.

Note:

The intent of advance asanas is not to show off, instead they are practiced when the body is simply capable of doing them. You need to take time mastering the more simple variations before practicing the more advanced poses. It might take years of consistent practice to achieve the ability to practice the advance variations. However, even with practice you might not get to the advance variations because of body conditions, age factor, or where your true interests lie. So please read your body as you encounter difficult postures, and always remember to gaze inward while you are holding the postures.

Vinyasa:

Vinyasa Left Side Down:

Exit from hanumanasana, step back to plank position and lean on your left hand and prepare for vinyasa left side down.

Now repeat vinyasa left side down one time (Figures: 14, 15, and 16).

Turn:

From vinyasa left side down, bring your right leg forward placing your right foot next to your left hand, which is holding the weight of your body, press the right foot into the floor and turn to the left 180 degrees.

Orientation:

Face the direction on the mat representing North.

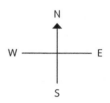

Asanas:

Eka Pada Sirsasana:

Eka: one; pada: foot; sirsa: head. It is leg behind the head posture.

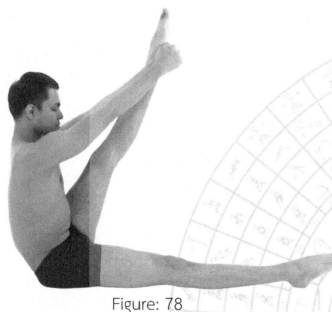

Figure: 78

There are many variations of leg behind head. Beginners should choose a variation from the first steps (Figures: 78, 79, 80). If you are an advance practitioner, choose a pose that is appropriate from the advance variations. You can warm-up with the initial steps as needed but spend the most time with one of the more challenging variations.

How to enter:

Step 1:

From your high lunge position after the turn, you will need to transit vinyasa to a seated position. Start by bringing your left arm under your left leg, float your legs up off the floor, bring your right thigh towards your chest, then straighten your right leg as you bring it through your arms. Now sit on the buttocks, your left leg is still behind the left shoulder,

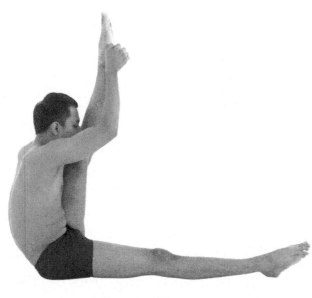

Figure: 79

ready for eka pada sirsasana (Figure: 80). If your hamstrings or lower back are weak, bring your left leg in front of you grabbing your left heel with both hands (Figure: 78). Gradually pull the leg towards the left shoulder (Figure: 79).

Step 2:

If you have enough flexibility in your left hip and hamstrings, then grab your left outer foot with your right hand bringing your leg behind your left shoulder (Figure: 80). Keep your knees straight, place your left hand on the floor, and lengthen your spine. At first your left sit bone might lift up, but through gradual practice both sit bones will rest on the floor.

Step 3:

Eka pada sirsasana has seven variations. If you are ready to put your foot behind your head, please choose one of the following seven

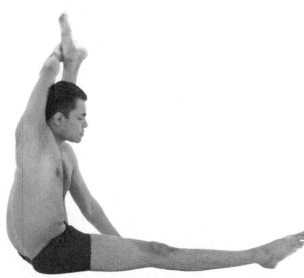

Figure: 80

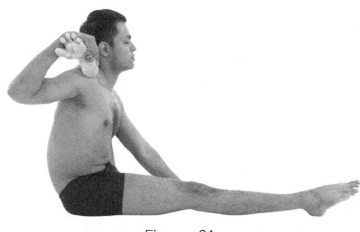

Figure: 81

variations. You do not need to do all of them.

Variation 1:

Flex your knee and hip. Externally rotate your left leg placing it behind your neck using your right hand. Keep holding your left leg, bend your spine forward slightly, and nudge your leg deep into the pose (Figure: 81). Relax your left leg, gradually lengthen your spine, and have a sense of slightly raising your neck. Try to look up to gain more resistance from the back of your neck. Stay for six breaths.

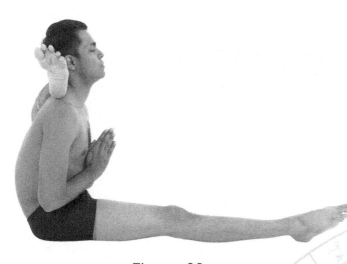

Figure: 82

Variation 2:

Follow the same steps as in variation 1 (Figure: 81). Once your head and neck can hold your leg, bring your palms together at the center of your heart in namaste mudra (Figure: 82). Stay for six breaths.

Variation 3:

Follow the same steps as in variation 1 (Figure: 81). After the left leg comes behind your neck, extend your right arm up and bind it on the left foot joining your hands together in namaste mudra on the lateral side of your torso (Figure: 83). Stay for six breaths.

141

Variation 4:

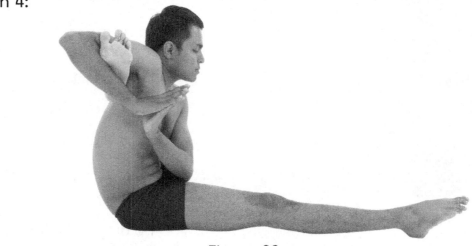

Figure: 83

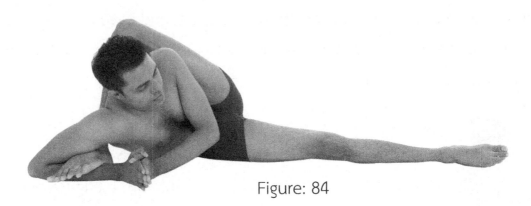

Figure: 84

Step 1:

Follow the same steps as in variation 3 (Figure: 83). Then lie down laterally onto your right side keeping your hands together in namaste mudra (Figure: 84).

Step 2:

Flex your right knee with the support of your left hand. Gently pull the right foot towards your left groin (Figure: 85).

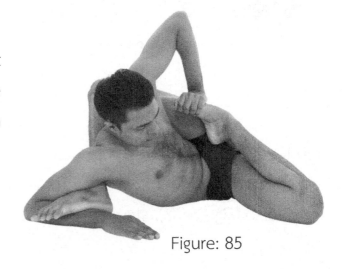

Figure: 85

142

Step 3:

Bind your right foot with your left elbow wrapping your right hand under your left hand (Figure 86). Avoid rushing your breath since your diaphragm and abdomen are contracting deeply. Lengthen your spine and allow space for your abdomen to expand and

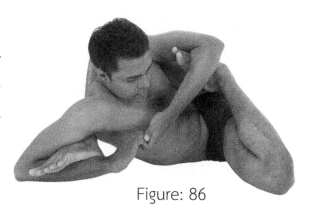

Figure: 86

breathe deeply from your lungs. The longer you hold this advance pose the more aware you should become of what is happening in the body. The asana might look attractive, but don't be seduced by it, rather allow yourself to practice regularly to bring more awareness into the physical sensations. Observe the rhythm of your breath until it feels effortless and graceful.

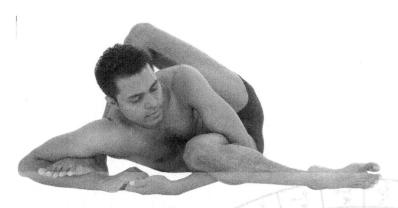

Figure: 87

Variation 5:

Follow the same steps for variation 4. Once you get to step 3 (Figure: 86), add the following variation. Flex your right hip and knee, bring your left arm under the right leg, and grab your right fingers with your left finger. Keep your head in line with your spine and avoid tilting it down (Figure: 87).

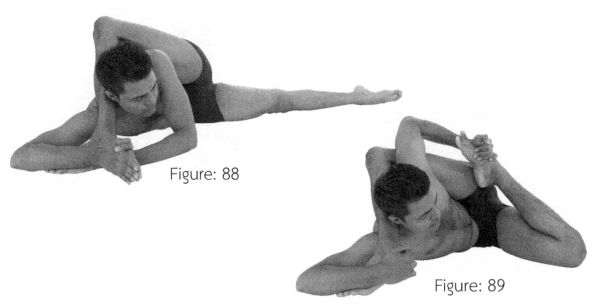

Figure: 88

Figure: 89

Variation 6:

This is an advance variation where you bind your left and right hands with the left foot on the floor in front of your right arm instead of behind. If you have mastered the previous variations of eka pada sirsasana, then these asanas become easier to access.

Follow the same steps from variation 4 and 5 except place the foot on the floor instead of having it on the right arm (Figure: 84 compared to Figure: 88; Figure: 85 compared to Figure: 89; Figure: 86 compared to Figure: 90; and Figure: 87 compared to Figure: 91). Also, place the hand in namaste mudra (Figure: 88 and 91).

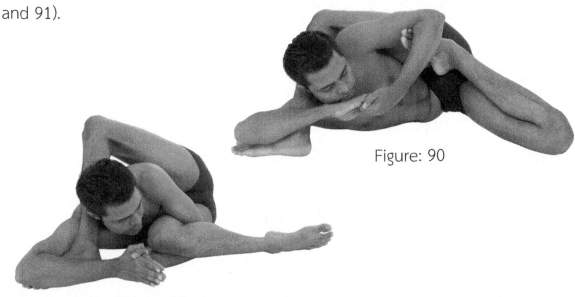

Figure: 90

Figure: 91

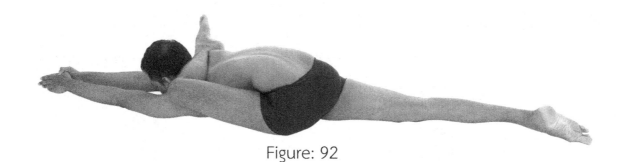

Figure: 92

Variation 7:

This is a complex variation in eka pada sirsasana. In order to attempt this posture, one needs to have deep external rotation of the hips and flexion of the spine. First follow the necessary steps for variation 2 (Figure: 82). Once your left leg comes behind your neck, then turn to your right and roll over into a plank-like pose. Gently lower the knee. Once your hip is open enough, tilt your head up pressing your chest to the floor. If you can manage to press your chest and chin to the floor, then bring your hands forward into anjali mudra (Figure: 92). Keep the back leg straight and active; stay for six breaths. To release, gently bring your hands on either side of your chest and push up. Then you can carefully release your leg from behind your head.

Note:

In the beginning stage, you can use your hands in chaturanga position and just drop your knee and forehead down, trying to stay for up to a minute. Once you progress, then rest your whole body on the floor.

With a consistent practice, your body will start to settle down in the poses. Each pose has its own beauty and grandeur to express gracefully. There are a wide range of eka pada sirsasana variations. Choose the pose you are ready for, practice carefully, and hold the pose for six breaths. When you are ready to release, gently remove the leg from behind your head.

Eka Pada Yoga Dandasana:

Eka: one; pada: foot; danda: staff. In this pose your foot is hooked under your armpit like a staff is kept to keep one in a meditative state.

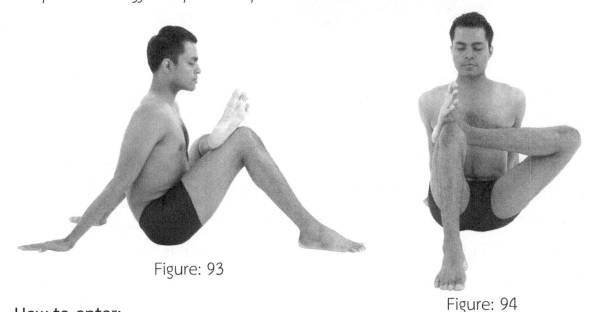

Figure: 93

Figure: 94

How to enter:

Step 1:

After releasing from eka pada sirsasana, sit with knees bent and feet on the floor. Lift your left foot and place your outer ankle on top of your right thigh close to the knee, creating a lateral rotation of your left hip joint. This will stretch your gluteus maximus and medius. Flex your left foot and place both hands behind you on the floor (Figures: 93 and 94).

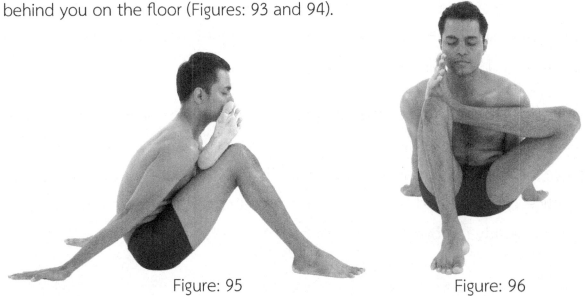

Figure: 95

Figure: 96

Step 2:

Once you are capable of placing your ankle on top of your thigh effortlessly, gently push your chest towards the inner left ankle while lengthening your spine (Figures: 95 and 96).

Step 3:

In this step you have to twist your torso, make sure there isn't any tension or irritation on the inner or outer sides of the knee.

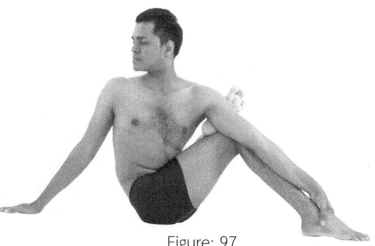

Figure: 97

As you exhale, keep the spine lengthening while you twist your torso to the right. Put your left foot in your right armpit, then grab the inner edge of your right foot with your left hand. Turn your head to the right (Figures: 97 and 98). Hold for six breaths.

Advance variation 1:

If your practice is getting deeper and you can easily catch your right foot with your left hand (Figure: 97), while exhaling lie down on your right side, bring your chin to the floor, and keep the right leg straight (Figure: 99). Remember to keep your left foot under your left armpit. If the foot is slippery it might slide down to your elbow, then the pose will not be effective at all. Once you hook your foot under the armpit firmly, then place your chin on the floor and direct your right

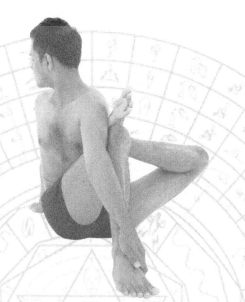

Figure: 98

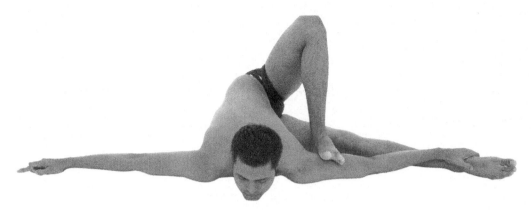

Figure: 99

arm to the side in line of your right shoulder. If you can do it fairy well, then see if you can grab your left shin with your right hand and press the chin down firmly (Figure: 100).

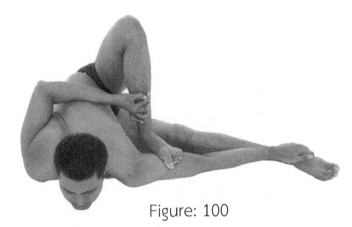

Figure: 100

Advance variation 2:

Step 1:

Unlike the previous variation, when you hook your left foot under the armpit, grab your left knee with your left hand. Keep your right leg straight, flex your torso forward, and elongate your spine. Now grab the outer edge of your right foot with your right hand (Figure: 101). Keep your right leg active and rest your right shoulder on top of your right leg, while placing your chin on the floor to help keep the spine in proper alignment.

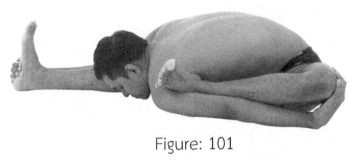

Figure: 101

Figure: 102

148

Step 2:

Bring your right arm behind your back in a medial rotation and grab your left fingers with your right hand (Figure: 102).

Advance variation 3:

Follow the same steps for variation 1 (Figure: 101), then extend your right hand over your head, release your left hand and medially rotate your left shoulder so you can bend your elbows. Your hands will be in a position as if you could tap on your own back. Wrap your left fingers with your right hand like two hooks (Figures: 103 and 104). Keep your spine and neck steady. Hold for six breaths.

Asanas have no limitations. Practice is a never ending journey, therefore play with the complex techniques when your body is ready. If you can overcome your fears, it is possible to access all of these asanas. If your body is not ready, then avoid the advance asanas and simply play with the basic asanas. You will still gain great benefits.

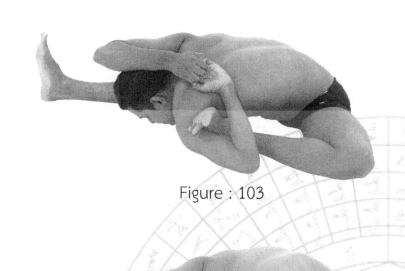

Figure : 103

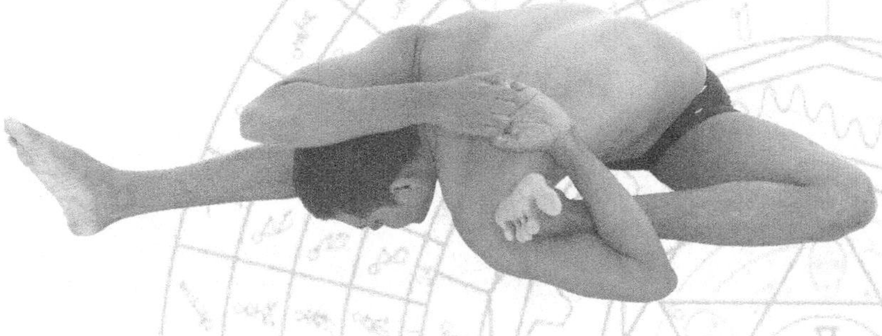

Figure : 104

Vinyasa:

Vinyasa Left Side Down:

After finishing eka pada yoga dandasana, step back to plank position and lean on your left hand and prepare for vinyasa left side down.

Now repeat vinyasa left side down one time (Figures: 14, 15, and 16).

Turn:

From vinyasa left side down, bring your right leg forward placing your right foot next to your left hand, which is holding the weight of your body, press the right foot into the floor and turn to the left 90 degrees.

Orientation:

Face the direction on the mat representing West.

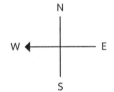

Asanas:

Eka Bhuja Kapotasana:

Eka: one; bhuja: arm; kapota: pigeon.

Pigeon pose is typically done with the legs, knees bent 90 degrees with a rotation of the hip. In Universal Yoga®, the same concept is used to activate the shoulder. This represents pigeon in the form of arms.

There are simple to advance variations of this pose. Pick the hardest variation that still allows you to stay effortlessly. Once you master one variation you can go to a more advance option.

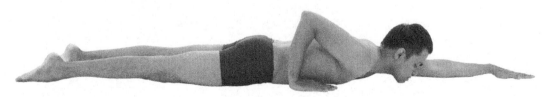

Figure: 105

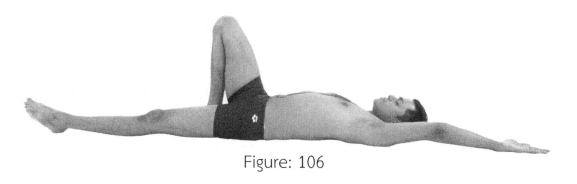

Figure: 106

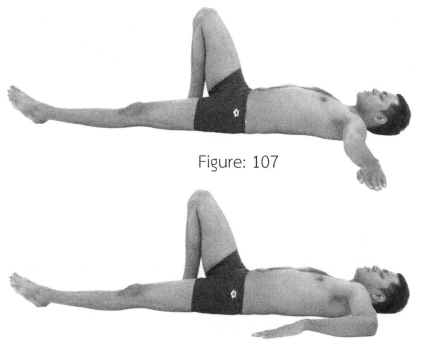

Figure: 107

Figure: 108

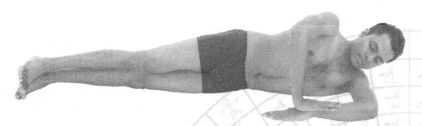

Figure: 109

How to enter:

Step 1:

Lie on your stomach directing your right hand overhead (Figure: 105). Roll over onto your buttocks, bend your right knee, and place your right foot on the floor (Figure: 106).

Step 2:

Stretch your right arm out to the side in line with your right shoulder, palm facing down (Figure: 107). Bend your right elbow 90 degrees, keeping your palm on the floor (Figure: 108).

Step 3:

Roll onto your right side while keeping the right shoulder on the floor. Press your left palm on top of your right wrist, raise your head up off the floor. Gently use the hips as a lever to turn towards the floor, stretching your right shoulder (Figure: 109).

This pose creates a deep medial rotation of the shoulder joint; avoid overdoing the pose.

Advance variation 1:

Follow the same steps as mentioned previously. If you have progressed in the range of motion at your shoulder, then place your left knee on the floor. Eventually rotate to get your abdomen on the floor with straight legs (Figure: 110).

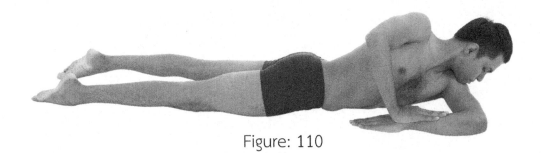

Figure: 110

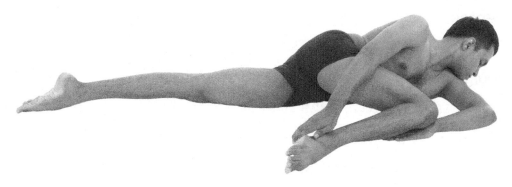

Figure: 111

Advance variation 2:

In this complex position, exhale as you place the left inner edge of your knee on top of your right palm. Without raising your right shoulder, grab the left outer heel with your left hand. Avoid hanging your head back; instead gently turn your head to face down towards the floor (Figure: 111). Keep the left leg straight and stay for six breaths.

As you inhale come out of the pose in the same order you entered. Then lay on your stomach.

Baddha Eka Bhuja Swastikasana:

Baddha: bound; eka: one; bhuja: arm; swastika: symbol of swastika.

The pose represents the swastika symbol with a bound variation, hence the name of the pose.

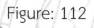

Figure: 112

153

How to enter:

Step 1:

Lie on your stomach, as you exhale cross your right arm under your throat to the left. Now medially rotate the right shoulder and keep your right elbow straight. Then bring your left arm next to the right thigh, press your left shoulder down towards the right forearm. Move your right leg to the right side in line with your right hip. Press your left shoulder further down toward the right forearm or floor (Figure: 112). Keep your left leg back and firmly pressed to the floor. Place your chin on the central plane of your spine. This pose stretches your shoulder girdle, latissimus dorsi, trapezius, and forearm.

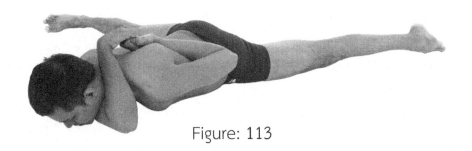

Figure: 113

Step 2:

Flex your right elbow and place your right palm on your back behind your right scapula. Now flex your left elbow and bring it behind your back to bind with your right fingers. Your shoulders medially rotate in this pose. Avoid choking your throat (Figure: 113). Stay for six deep breaths. Then exhale to release the pose the same way you entered.

Vinyasa:

Vinyasa Left Side Down:

After exiting baddha eka bhuja swastikasana, step back to plank position and lean on your left hand and prepare for vinyasa left side down.

Now repeat vinyasa left side down one time (Figures: 14, 15, and 16).

Turn:

From vinyasa left side down, bring your right leg forward placing your right foot next to your left hand, which is holding the weight of your body. Press the right foot into the floor and turn to the left 180 degrees.

Orientation:

Face the direction on the mat representing East.

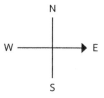

Asanas:

Eka Bhuja Kapotasana 2:

Eka: one; bhuja: arms; kapota: pigeon. This is one of the many variations of one arm pigeon pose.

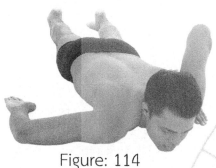

Figure: 114

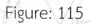

Figure: 115

How to enter:

Step 1:

Lie on your stomach, direct your right arm to the side in line with your right shoulder. Now bend your right elbow, internally rotate your right shoulder and place your right fingers facing backwards (Figure: 114). Raise your right elbow a little bit higher than your right shoulder in line with your right ear (Figure: 115). Now roll onto your right hip, bend your knees keeping them hip distance apart. Place the sole of your feet firmly on the floor. If the pose is easy, then rest your buttocks on the floor.

Step 2:

Now bring your left hand back and interlace it with your right hand (Figure: 116 and 117). Stay for six deep breaths and exit from the pose.

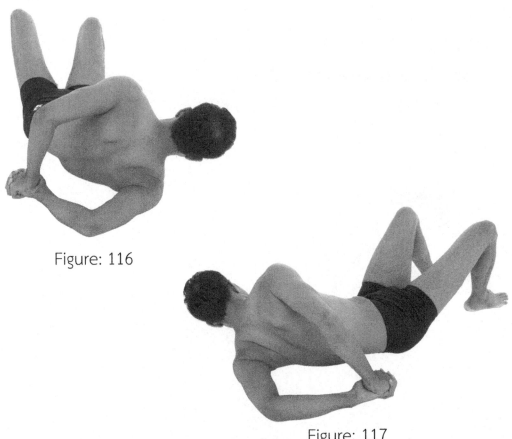

Figure: 116

Figure: 117

Eka Bhuja Kapotasana 3:

Eka: one; bhuja: arm, kapota: pigeon. Here is another variation of an arm position which resembles pigeon pose as done with the legs.

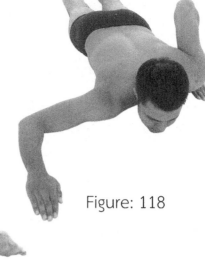

Figure: 118

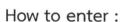

Figure: 119

How to enter :

Step 1:

Lay on your stomach, direct your right arm to the side, bend your elbow 90 degrees, keep your fingers facing forward, and your palm down (Figure: 118). Move your elbow a little higher than your shoulder. (Figure: 119).

Step 2:

Roll onto your right hip, place your left palm on the floor in front of your chest, bend your knees up to the level of your hips, and rest the side of your head on the floor (Figure: 120). Now bring your left foot into half lotus position. Push your left palm on the inside of your left knee, gently push your left knee away to firmly press

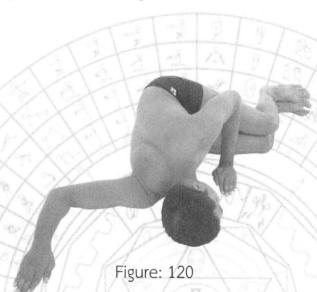

Figure: 120

157

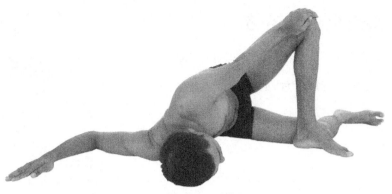

Figure: 121

your right shoulder to the floor. Simultaneously, direct your left shoulder back toward the line of your right elbow (Figure: 121). This creates an incredible external rotation of your right shoulder. If you have stiff shoulders, apply gentle pressure or just place the left hand on the floor. If accessible, press into your palms and gently lift your head up. Notice the sensation around the shoulder. If it is painful or you have any nerve impingements or a frozen shoulder, don't overstretch. Stay for six breaths, then as you exhale release the pose.

Advance variation 1:

If you are ready to advance the pose, place your right foot on top of your left thigh and bring your left leg over the right thigh into full lotus position. Keep your left foot on the floor, place your right hand on the inside of your left knee keeping the elbow straight, and rest your head on the floor (Figure: 122).

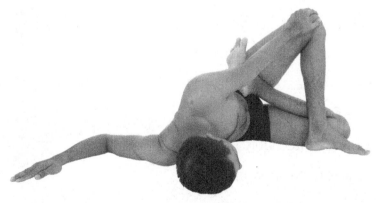

Figure: 122

Vinyasa:

Vinyasa Left Side Down:

After exiting eka bhuja kapotasana, step back to plank position and lean on your left hand and prepare for vinyasa left side down.

Now repeat vinyasa left side down one time (Figures: 14, 15, and 16).

Turn:

From vinyasa left side down, bring your right leg forward placing your right foot next to your left hand which is holding the weight of your body. Press the right foot into the floor and turn to the left 90 degrees.

Orientation:

Face the direction on the mat representing North.

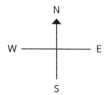

Asanas:

Ardha Chandrasana

Ardha: half; chandra: moon. This pose represents the half standing moon position.

How to enter:
Step 1:

Stand with both feet together, raise your arms up over your head catching the back of your right wrist with your left hand, and keep your right hand in mushti mudra. As you inhale, lengthen your spine. As you exhale, arch up and over to the left. This helps to elongate your upper back, neck, and spine.

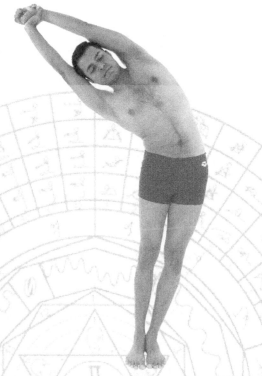

Figure: 123

159

Keep your chest lifting up, pelvis in neutral position, and legs straight. Pull the right arm towards the left side keeping your neck neutral. Keep your face forward, nose is neither pointing upward nor facing downward. Both legs are firm and steady (Figure: 123). Avoid bending the knees. Stay for six breaths, then release.

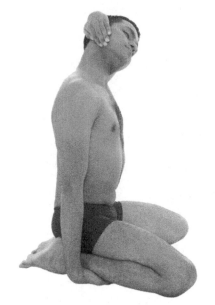

Figure: 124

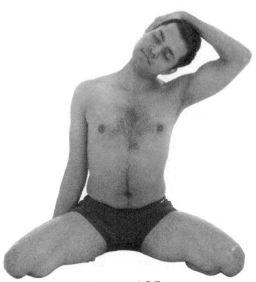

Figure: 125

Parsva Grivasana:

Parsva: half; griva: neck.

How to enter:
Step 1:

Sit in vajrasana with your knees wide, toes together, and rest your sit bones on the heels. As you exhale, grab your right shin with your right hand and sweep your left hand over your head to reach your right cheek or ear. Move your left ear toward your left shoulder (Figure: 125). This pose stretches the trapezius, levator scapula, and sternocleidomastoid. It is an important asana for stretching your neck deeply and helps to prepare your upper back for deep backbends. Stay for six breaths, then exhale and release from the pose.

Vinyasa:

Vinyasa Abdominal Down:

After exiting parsva grivasana, step back to plank pose. As you exhale, lower your body to chaturanga dandasana. Inhale and arch your torso up and back into urdhva mukha svanasana. Exhale and tuck your toes under and lift your hips high into adho mukha svanasana (Figures: 9, 10, and 11).

Turn:

From adho mukha svanasana (Figure: 11) jump legs wide and turn left 90 degrees.

Orientation:

Face the direction on the mat representing West.

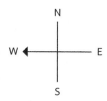

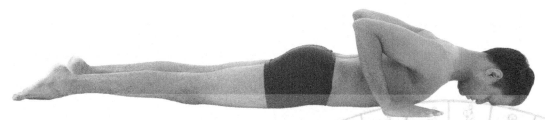

Figure: 126

Asanas:

Bhujangasana:

Bhujanga: snake or serpent. In this pose, your body moves into a deep backbend with your head facing up to look like a cobra.

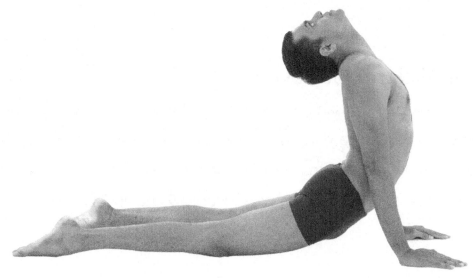

Figure: 127

How to enter:

Step 1:

Lie on your stomach, place your palms next to your chest, toes pointing back in plantar flexion, and feet hip distance apart (Figure: 126). If your back is flexible enough, keep your toes together and stretch your legs back firmly.

As you inhale press your palms down, lift your chest up, and straighten your arms into a vertical position. Arch your neck backwards (Figure: 127). Breathe

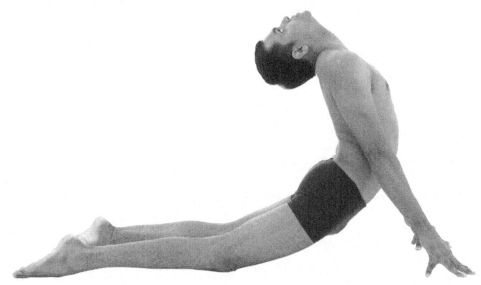

Figure: 128

slowly and avoid holding your breath. Do not lean on your hands into your lower back, rather raise your chest up and protract your shoulder back. Hold for six breaths.

Advance variation 1:

To deepen the pose, come onto your finger tips. Be sure that your fingers are strong enough to hold up the weight of

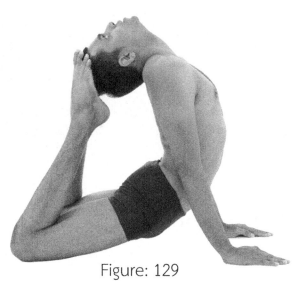
Figure: 129

your torso, then arch back further without creating any tension. Keep your face relaxed and breathe comfortably (Figure: 128). Stay for six breaths. Release by lowering down and resting your forehead on the floor.

Advance variation 2:

When you are able to perform full bhujangasana without any effort, then you can add more complex positions to deepen your backbend.

Start with the steps for advance variation 1, then bend your knees and bring your feet towards your head (Figure: 129). When that is accessible, place your toes under the back of your head (Figure: 130).

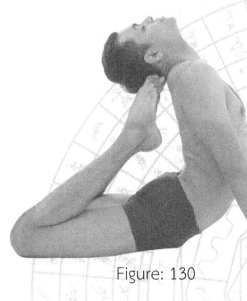
Figure: 130

163

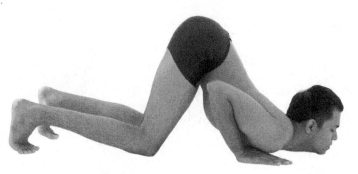

Figure: 131

Marjariasana:

Marjari: cat. This pose resembles a cat stretching.

How to enter:

Step 1:

Lie on your stomach with your chin on the floor and bring your hands on either side of your chest. Now exhale and walk your knees forward lifting your hips. Position your knees at a 90 degree angle under your hips. Keep your chin on the floor backbending your neck (Figure: 131). Stay for six long breaths.

Advance variation 1:

Step 1:

If your upper back is flexible and you are able to breathe freely, then stretch your arms forward, keeping them shoulder distance apart with your palms facing down. Your chest might come off the floor, so activate your upper back to press it down deeply to find a good range of motion. Do not hold yourself up with your hands, instead use your upper back and neck muscles to stretch down deeply (Figure: 132).

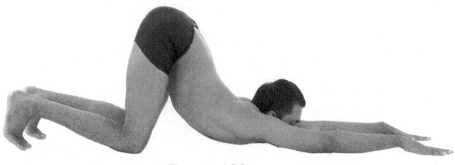

Figure: 132

Vinyasa:

Vinyasa Abdominal Down:

After exiting marjiriasana, step back to plank pose. Exhale while lowering your body into chaturanga dandasana. Inhale and arch your torso up and back into urdhva mukha svanasana. Exhale and tuck your toes under and lift your hips high into adho mukha svanasana (Figures: 9, 10, and 11).

Turn:

From adho mukha svanasana (Figure: 11) jump legs wide and turn left 90 degrees.

Orientation:

Face the direction on the mat representing South.

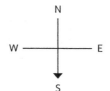

Vinyasa:

Chakra Vinyasa - Somersault Forward:

There are two vinyasas in this set, this second one is a somersault forward which is called a chakra vinyasa.

Step your legs together, bend your knees, and keep your toes tucked under. Now place your palms on the floor and flex your neck bringing your chin toward your chest (Figure: 133). As you exhale, bend forward and place the back of your head onto the floor. As you round your neck further to the floor, gently raise your hips in the air (Figure: 134). Remember to keep your neck relaxed. Now using the strength from your legs and arms, roll forward. Place your upper back on the floor (Figure: 135) then roll forward and sit (Figure: 136).

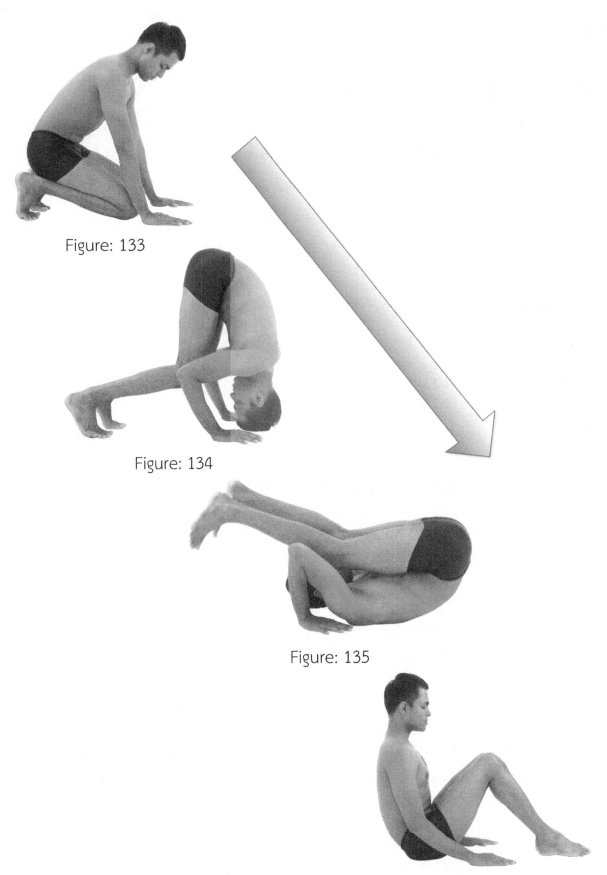

Figure: 133

Figure: 134

Figure: 135

Figure: 136

Parivrtta Janu Sirsasana:

Parivrtta: revolved; janu: knee; sirsa: head. This pose is revolved head to knee pose.

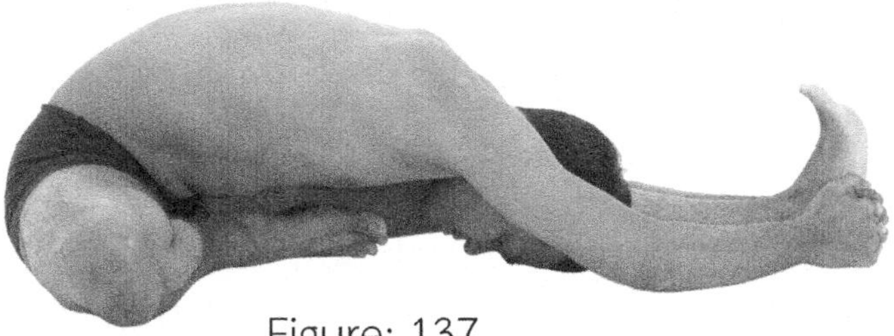

How to enter:

Step 1:

Start by sitting with straight legs,

Figure: 137

then bend your left knee and externally rotate the thigh at your hip. Place your left foot next to your right inner thigh, while keeping your hips fairly square. With your right leg straight, bend your torso forward and catch your right heel with your hands. As you elongate your spine, you will create a deeper stretch for your back and hamstrings. Lower your right shoulder to your right leg, letting your head rest on the floor (Figure: 137). This keeps your spine properly aligned. Avoid lifting your sit bones off the floor.

Step 2:

If your knee is comfortable and your hamstrings are fairly open, then grab your left knee with your right hand, and grab the outer edge of your right foot with your left hand. Ground your left sit bone and turn your head to gaze up toward the ceiling in a deep twist (Figure: 138). This twist gives a deep stretch for your quadratus lumborum and abdomen region. Balance the level of inhalation and exhalation at equal ratios. When confident in this pose, close your eyes and detach from your body, leaving an imprint of your internal sensations and feel the control and sense of awareness within you. Hold for six breaths then release.

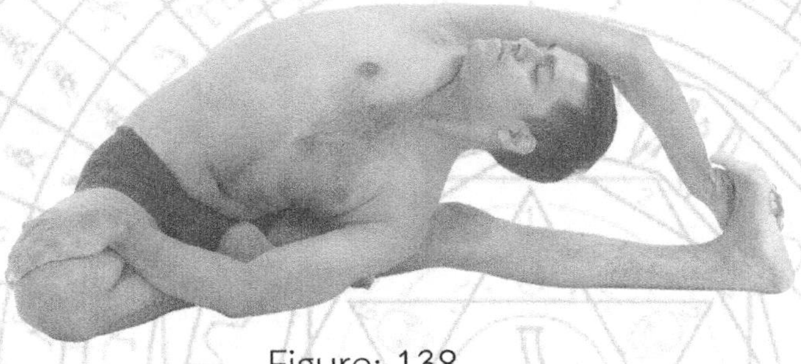

Figure: 138

167

Ardha Nirlamba Sarvangasana:

Ardha: half; nirlamba: unsupported; sarvanga: whole body. This pose is an unsupported shoulderstand.

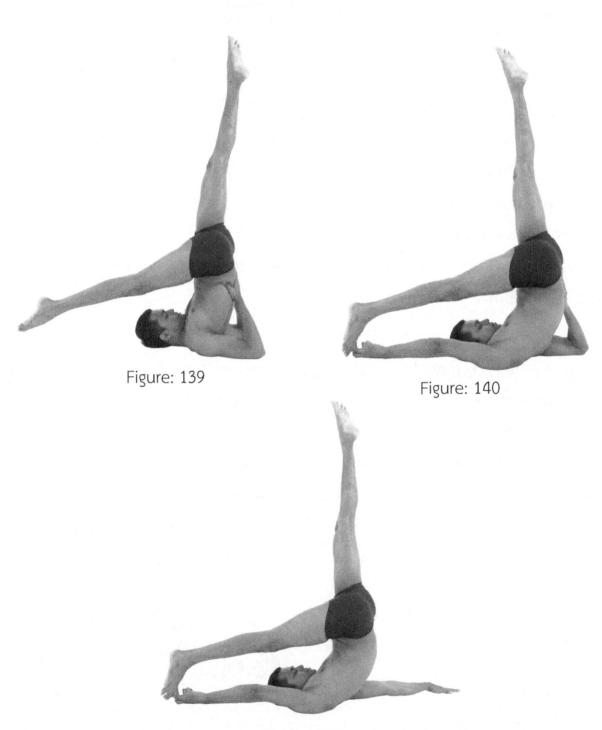

Figure: 139

Figure: 140

Figure: 141

How to enter:

Step 1:

After you release from parivrtta janu sirsasana, lie down on your back. As you inhale, lift your pelvis and legs up using your abdomen muscles to bring your body into a vertical position.

Keep your neck in the central plane of your spine. Bend your elbows and catch your hips or mid back with your palms. Firmly press your upper arms into the floor, elbows in line with your shoulders. Since Universal Yoga® practice is about creating balance throughout the body, and by now your shoulders are more open from the previous shoulder stretches, you will probably feel that the shoulders responded well to bringing your elbows closer. Now bring your right leg towards the floor over your head placing your right toes on the floor. Keep your left leg straight up to the sky, and slightly rotate your left femur bone inward, toes pointing upward into plantar flexion position (Figure: 139).

Step 2:

Once you have your balance and your body is in a straight line, bring your right hand over your head and grab your right foot (Figure: 140). When your balance is under control again, release the left arm straight down on the floor (Figure: 141). Slightly lengthen the chin to create a small space between your chin and chest. This will elongate the neck and spine. Avoid locking the chin. This practice can be done by locking the chin as well during specific energetic practices, however since this practice is an asana practice, bandhas are not used to lock in. Rather be conscious on how to attain balance in the posture. Hold for six to eight long breaths.

Vinyasa:

Ardha Chakra Vinyasa - Half Somersault Backward:

From ardha nirlamba sarvangasana, place your hands by your head with your fingers pointing towards your shoulders. Roll backwards by pressing your toes on the floor simultaneously pressing your palms firmly under your shoulders, and lifting your hips up over your head (Figure: 144). When you roll back, use momentum and the strength of your hands, legs, and the back of your neck to roll backwards; then rest your knees on the floor (Figure: 145). Push into your hands to come up (Figure: 146).

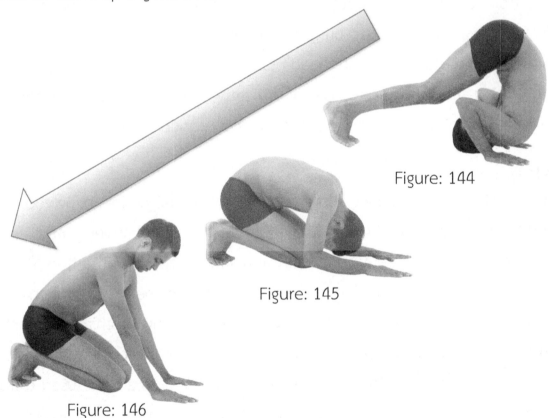

Figure: 144

Figure: 145

Figure: 146

Turn:

After ardha chakra vinyasa, jump legs wide, then turn left 90 degrees.

Orientation:

Face the direction on the mat representing East.

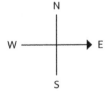

170

Asanas:

Ardha Matsyendrasana:

Ardha: half; matsya: fish. This pose is dedicated to sage Matsyendranath, hence the name.

There are many variations of ardha matsyendrasana. While you are practicing the full sequence for energetic results, choose one variation of the pose and hold. Avoid trying to practice all of the variations during a single practice. Beginners should practice the simpler variation. If you choose an advance pose, be sure that you are not struggling or forcing the pose.

How to enter:

Step 1:

After the vinyasa and turning left 90 degrees to face East, your left foot will be facing forward. Now cross your right knee to the outside of your left ankle and sit on the floor with your left foot flat. Your right leg is now on the floor in an external rotation of the hip; your right foot is next to your left outer hip. Keep your pelvis symmetrical. Next, inhale and raise your right arm up, exhale and bend your elbow, place your right arm across your left knee (Figures: 147 and 148). This is an optimal pose for beginners to stay in and hold for six breaths.

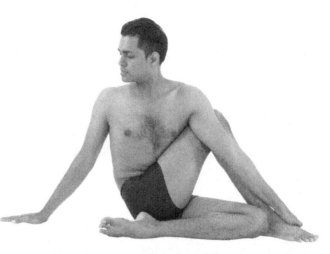

Figure: 147

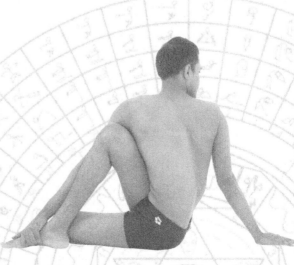

Figure: 148

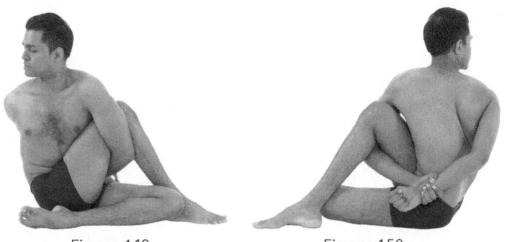

Figure: 149   Figure: 150

Step 2:

If you are ready to add on, you will bind your left leg. Start by internally rotating your right shoulder, exhale and bring your right arm behind your back. The shoulder rotation can help facilitate your right arm binding around your left leg deeply so you can clasp your right wrist with your left hand. Avoid leaning backwards, keep the spine straight, and turn your head towards the line of the left shoulder (Figures: 149 and 150).

This is a deep spinal twist which helps to activate the lumbar and thoracic vertebra and massages the abdomen through deep breaths. Do not hold the breath, keep the breath rhythmic, stay for six to ten long breaths, and then release.

Advance variation 1:

Step 1:

Follow the previous steps of ardha matsyendrasana, then flex your right elbow deeper and raise your left arm up into extension, externally rotate the left shoulder, and flex your elbow. Now bring your left hand behind your back to clasp your right fingers. As you bind the hands, gently protract the scapula down which helps to engage the shoulder girdle and take pressure off the shoulders (Figures: 151 and 152).

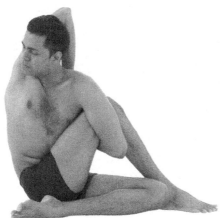

Figure : 151

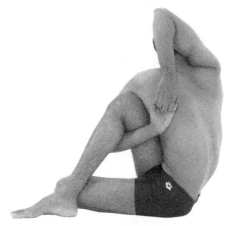

Figure : 152

This is an advance variation; do not jump into advance movements without mastering the earlier stages. This variation puts a strong emphasis on the shoulders, particularly because internally rotating the shoulder activates the posterior deltoid, rotator cuff muscles, and teres major. The shoulder also being in an extension position activates the anterior region of the deltoids, pectoralis minor, rhomboids, and scapula.

Advance variation 2:

Step 1:

Sit on the floor, place your right foot over your left thigh into half lotus pose. Now flex your left knee, bring your foot flat on the floor, and place it next to your right knee. Your right foot is aligned within your lower abdomen, move your belly out of the way, exhale while hooking your right arm across your left knee, and grab your left foot (Figure: 153).

Step 2:

If possible, bring your left foot across your right knee putting it flat on the floor. Hook your right arm across your left knee and grab your foot. Place your left hand behind your left hip which will help you avoid leaning back. Gently turn your head back towards the line of your left shoulder (Figure: 154).

In this variation there is more emphasis on the knee and hips. If your hips are quite mobile then this pose will be accessible. The right leg is in deep external rotation at the hip, whereas your left leg rotates internally which goes beyond the movement of adduction. Balance the alignment between your hips and shoulders, avoid rupturing your meniscus on the right side of your inner knee joint. This pose activates the gluteus maximus, minimus, and medius. It also provides a deep twist in the lumbar and thoracic spine.

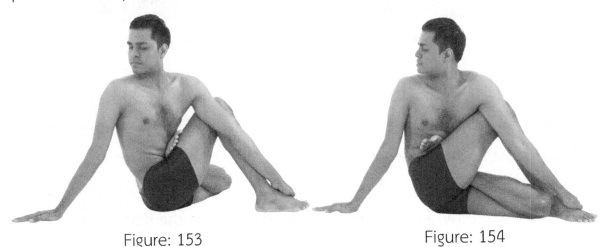

Figure: 153   Figure: 154

Parivrtta Grivasana:

Parivrtta: revolve; griva: neck.

How to enter:

Step 1:

Sit on the floor with your knees hip distance apart and bent at 60 degrees. Bend your elbows and place them on your knees. Spin your left fingers to face left keeping your palm facing up. Turn your head to the left and place your left hand under your right cheek. Keep your head in line with your spine (Figures: 155 and 156). Now bring your right hand behind the back of your head (Figure: 157). Apply gentle pressure with your hands to deeply twist your neck to the left (Figure: 158), but avoid over twisting as it could lead to injury. The right pressure can give effective results. Stay for six breaths, then release.

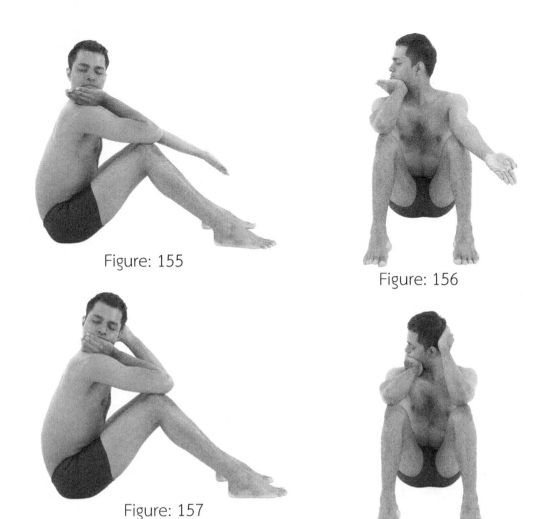

Figure: 155

Figure: 156

Figure: 157

Vinyasa:

Figure: 158

Chakra Vinyasa - Somersault Backward:

After you exit from parivrtta grivasana, sit on the floor with your knees bent (Figure: 159). As you exhale, tuck your chin towards your chest, roll backwards (Figure: 160), press your toes on the floor simultaneously pressing your palms firmly under your shoulders, and lift your hips up over your head (Figure: 161). When you roll back, use momentum and the strength of your hands, legs, and the back of your neck to roll backwards, then rest your knees on the floor (Figure: 162). Push into your hands to come up (Figure: 163).

Orientation:

Face the direction on the mat representing East.

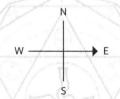

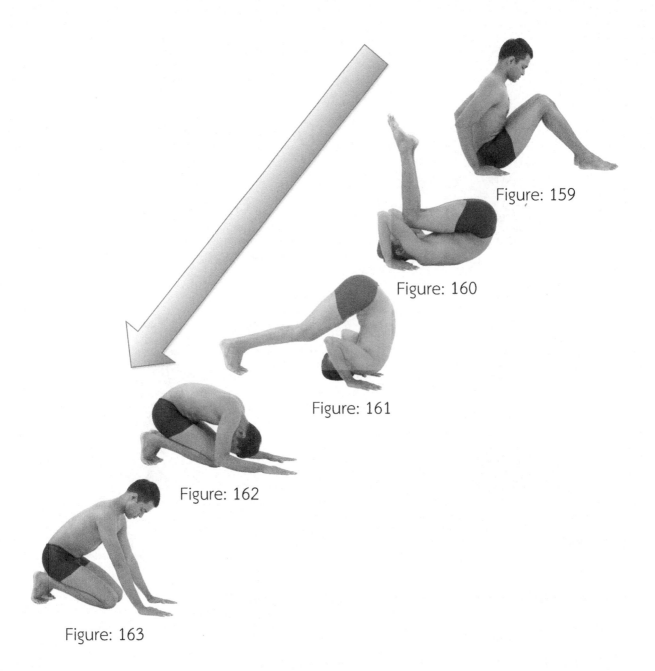

Figure: 159

Figure: 160

Figure: 161

Figure: 162

Figure: 163

Pranayama:

Sitali Chandra Bhedana:

This is a combination of sitali and chandra bhedana pranayama.

How to enter:

Sit in padmasana (lotus posture) or another comfortable seated position. Place your left hand into jnana mudra keeping your palm facing up on your thigh.

176

Bring your right palm up to your face (Figure: 164) and place your fingers on your forehead and your thumb by your right nostril. Curl your tongue and bring the tip of the tongue to your lower lip and keep your lips open slightly. As you inhale, breathe through your mouth until the lungs are filled. Now close your mouth and use your thumb to close your right nostril. As you exhale, breathe out slowly through your left nostril only, keeping the tip of the tongue on the roof of your mouth behind the front teeth. This is one round, repeat six times, then relax.

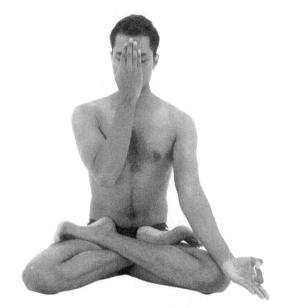

Figure: 164

Stillness:

Awareness:

Padmasana (lotus posture) or other comfortable seated position.

How to enter:

After finishing sitali chandra bhedana, sit in padmasana (Figure: 165) or any comfortable seated position. Close your eyes, relax your hands, experience the sensation of your internal layers within your subtle body. Stay for one to two minutes.

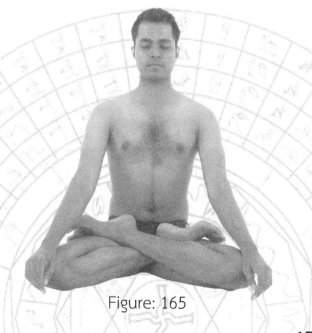

Figure: 165

Completion of First Side:

You have finished one side of the practice. You have created an energy diagonal shift from left leg to right arm. The diagonal shift of energy includes all asanas, vinyasas, turns on the mat, and pranayamas. This completes the first side.

Mirror Reflect the Sequence on the Opposite Side:

The same sequence will be repeated on the other side to complete the second diagonal cross from right leg to left arm. You will need to mirror reflect the previous set in all of the asanas, vinyasas, turns on the mat and pranayamas. This will balance the energy diagonal which resembles a cross line shift of energy in your body.

Start with vinyasa abdominal down (Page: 103), once you jump your legs wide you will turn 90 degrees to the right. All of the turns for this round will be to the right. When doing vinyasa side down, previously you did all of them with the left side facing down. Now you will practice with the right side down.

Note:

To keep the number of pages in this book manageable, the mirror reflection is not described or shown in detail. So simply repeat the sequence, just use right leg when the directions say left leg, and use left arm when the directions say right arm. At the end when you get back to the chakra vinyasa - somersault backward (Page: 178), go right to sitali surya bhedana pranayama (Page: 181).

Pranayama:

Sitali Surya Bhedana:

This is a combination of sitali and surya bhedana pranayama.

How to enter:

Sit in padmasana (lotus posture) or any comfortable seated position. Place your right hand into jnana mudra keeping your palm facing up on your thigh. Bring your left palm up to your face (Figure: 164) and place your fingers on your forehead and your thumb by your left nostril. Curl your tongue and bring the tip of the tongue to your lower lip, and keep your lips open slightly. As you inhale, breathe through your mouth until the lungs are filled. Now close your mouth and use your thumb to close your left nostril. As you exhale, breathe out slowly through your right nostril only, keeping the tip of the tongue on the roof of your mouth behind the front teeth. This is one round, repeat six times, then relax.

Stillness:

Awareness:

Padmasana (lotus posture) or other comfortable seated position.

How to enter:

After finishing sitali suyra bhedana, sit in padmasana (Figure: 165) or any comfortable seated position. Close your eyes, relax your hands, experience the sensation of your internal layers within your subtle body. Stay for one to two minutes.

Completion of Second Side:

You have created an energy diagonal shift from right leg to left arm. The diagonal shift of energy includes all asanas, vinyasas, turns on the mat, and pranayamas. This completes the second side.

Continue to the next part of the sequence.

Vinyasa:

Vinyasa Abdominal Down:

After exiting from awareness pose, uncross your legs, place your palms on the floor and exhale while jumping back into chaturanga dandasana. Do one vinyasa abdominal down (Figures: 9, 10 and 11).

From adho mukha svanansa (Figure: 11) jump your legs wide onto the transversal mat and stand up.

Orientation:

Face the direction on the mat representing East.

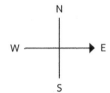

Asanas:

Pada Ardha Stupa Bhuja Garudasana:

Pada: leg; ardha: half; stupa: shape of a stupa; bhuja: arm; garuda: eagle

How to enter:

Step 1:

After jumping your legs wide from downward dog position, stand up and bend your left knee 90 degrees, keeping it in line with your second toe. Keep your right foot flat or flex it lifting your toes to the sky. Your left heel should line up with your right heel. Keep your spine

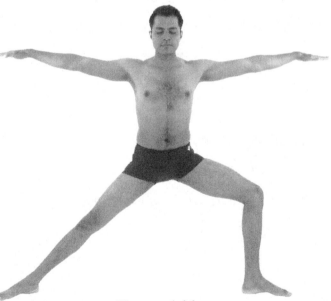

Figure: 166

straight and avoid sticking your sit bones out. Your hips should be in a neutral position. This asana demands incredible strength in your quadriceps. Ground your feet with your weight evenly distributed into both legs. Find your center of gravity in this asymmetrical asana. Once you maintain balance then bring your arms to the side in line with your shoulders (Figure: 166).

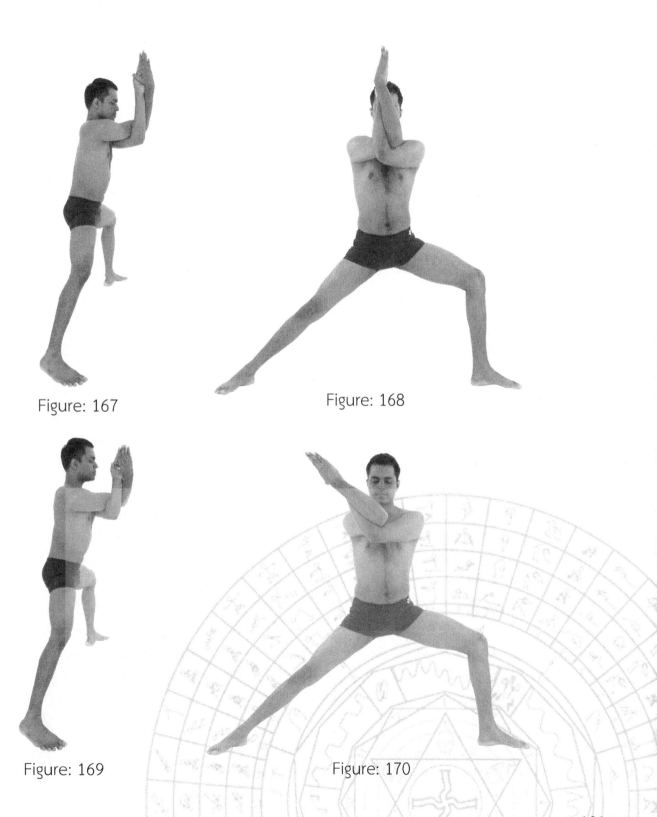

Figure: 167

Figure: 168

Figure: 169

Figure: 170

Step 2:

Cross your right arm over the left arm, bend your elbows, and bind the arms keeping your hands together in prayer position (Figures: 167 and 168). As you inhale retract your scapula, connecting the arms into the shoulder sockets. Then allow the back of the shoulders to broaden deeply. Now as you exhale, move

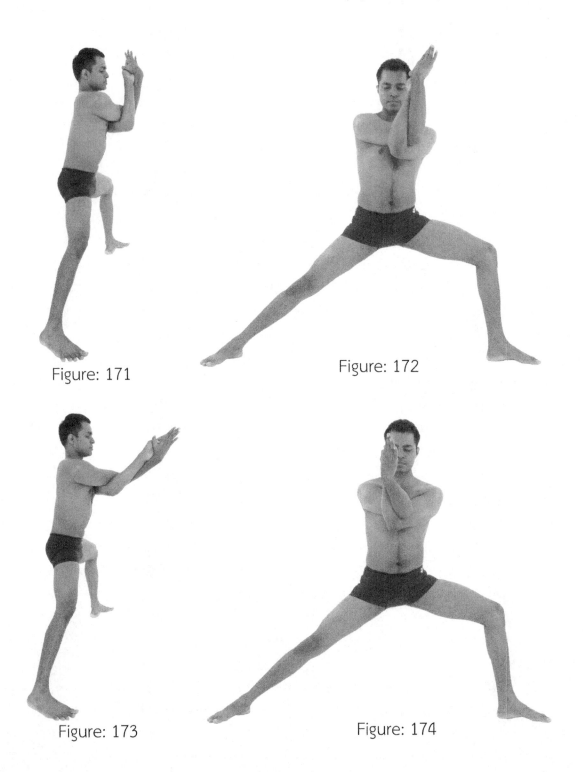

Figure: 171

Figure: 172

Figure: 173

Figure: 174

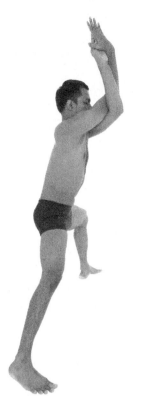

Figure: 175

your arms to the left (Figures: 169 and 170), pause for a few seconds, as you inhale return back to the center. Exhale while moving your arms to the right and pause (Figures: 171 and 172), as you inhale return back to the center. As you exhale move your arms down and pause (Figures: 173 and 174), inhale and return to the center. Exhale while moving your arms up and pause (Figure: 175), as you inhale return back to the center and release. During each move, stay for a few seconds, overall hold this pose for at least four long breaths.

Mirror reflection to your right side:
Repeat pada ardha stupa bhuja garudasana on your right side.

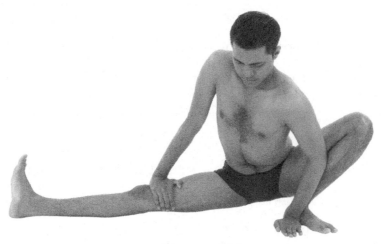

Figure: 176

Parshva Eka Padasana:

Parshva: side; eka: one; pada: leg

How to enter:

From pada ardha stupa bhuja garudasana, bend your left knee lowering your hips down, put your left elbow on your left inner knee, and keep your right leg out to the right side. Place your left palm on the floor with your fingers facing forward. Now gently push your left thigh back with the support of your left bent elbow. Place your right palm on your right thigh above the knee and press down. Be mindful with your right knee, it is easy to put too much pressure on the knee joint. While pressing on your right thigh, keep your right elbow straight (Figure: 176). Here the right leg is used as a lever to stretch your left hip and thigh deeply.

There are many variations to this pose. In the beginning, choose this easier variation until you have loosened up your hips, gluteus, gracillis, adductor magnus, and pectineus.

Advance variations 1:

When you are ready to add on, bend your left elbow, internally rotate your shoulder, extend your right arm over your head, bend your right elbow, and reach your fingers towards your scapula. Now clasp your hands (Figure: 177). Place your left elbow next to your left inner thigh. As you exhale, gently push your left leg away from your body. Now bend your torso towards the line of your right leg and bring your head towards the floor (Figure: 178). This particular movement will give your left hip a deep stretch.

In this advance variation, the element of shoulder work comes into play. You need to bind your arms behind your back instead of pressing into your leg. If you have any shoulder problems, such as an impingement or frozen shoulder, then please avoid this variation with the arms.

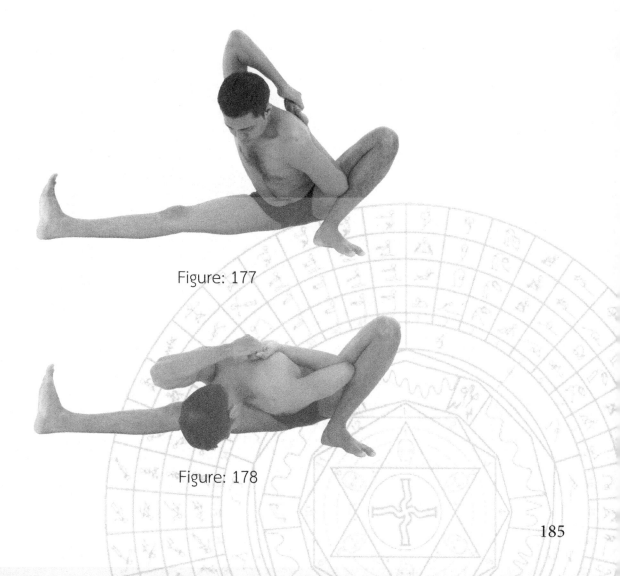

Figure: 177

Figure: 178

Advance variation 2:

This is a very advanced variation and body proportions play a major role. If your arms are long, your shoulders will elevate high. If the arms are equal with the proportion of your legs, then you can retract the scpaula fairly well.

From pada ardha stupa bhuja garudasana, lower the hips further down and lift your right foot up in dorsi flexion, standing on your right heel. Now place your left palm on your left thigh and right palm on your right thigh. Push on your legs with your straight arms and flex your body forward into the longitudinal plane (Figure: 179). This is a strong pose to build up your quadriceps, adductors, and soleus.

Hold any one of the pose variations for six long breaths.

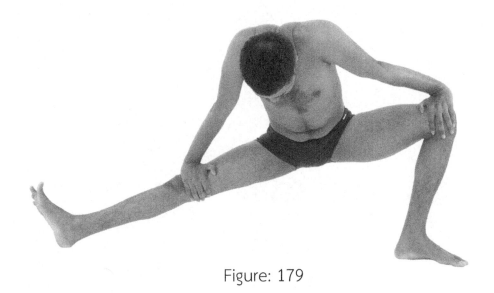

Figure: 179

Mirror reflection to your right side:

Repeat parshva eka padasana on your right side.

Stupasana:

Resembles the shape of a Buddhist stupa.

How to enter:

Stand with wide legs, turn your toes out 45 degrees, exhale while bending your knees, and lower your pelvis until your thighs are parallel with the floor. Lengthen your spine, avoid over arching your lower back, and slightly firm and pull in your abdomen. Your back and neck will be erect and neutral. Now inhale and lift your arms out to the side in line with your shoulders. Put your hands in mushti mudra keeping your palms facing down. Once you find your balance, close your eyes, and gaze internally for six breaths (Figure: 180). Exhale and release from the pose.

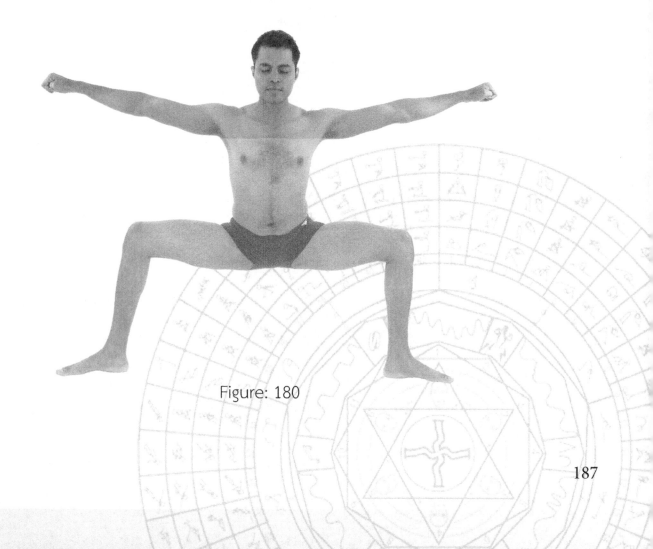

Figure: 180

Dwi Bhujasana:

Dwi: two; bhuja: arm. This pose stretches your biceps and forearms.

How to enter:

Release from stupasana and jump your leg together. Separate your feet hip width apart, squat down and place your hands on the floor. Turn your palms to face backwards so your fingers face your toes. Place your knees on your right upper arms above the elbows (Figure: 181). Reach the maximum level of your stretch, but don't push too hard with your knees. Hold for six breaths.

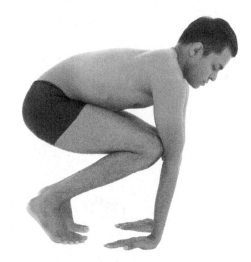

Figure: 181

Vinyasa:

Vinyasa Abdominal Down

Release from dwi bhujasana, step back to plank pose. Do one vinyasa abdominal down (Figures: 9, 10 and 11).

From adho mukha svanansa (Figure: 11) jump your legs wide onto the transversal mat.

Orientation:

Face the direction on the mat representing East.

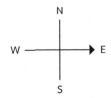

Asanas:

Samakonasana:

Sama: equal; kona: angle.

There are beginner to advance variations of samakonasa. In the beginning stages of your practice, it is safe to practice the easier variation. After exiting samakonasana, you will be doing the next asana, pada anupradhastasana, which is an asymmetrical asana. So, once you finish pada anupradhastasana on the left side, you will return back and repeat samakonasana. When you repeat a pose, the body tends to be more open, so you can go deeper. When you release from samakonasana, you will be repeating pada anupradhastasana but on the right side.

How to enter:

Step 1:

Exhale and bend your torso forward, place your hands on the floor, and spread your legs as wide apart as you can. Keep your legs firm and your feet flat on the floor (Figure: 182).

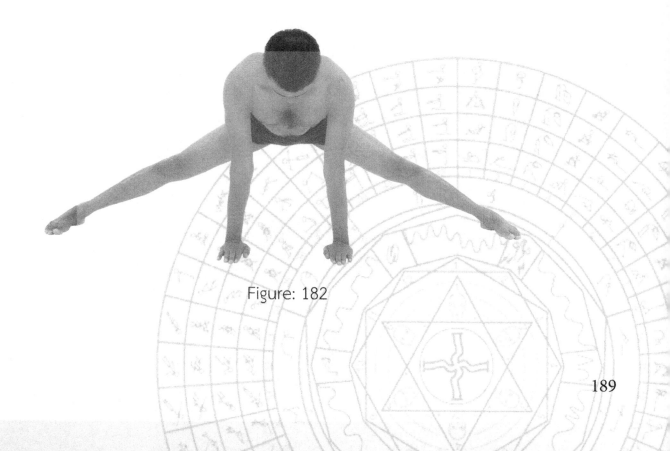

Figure: 182

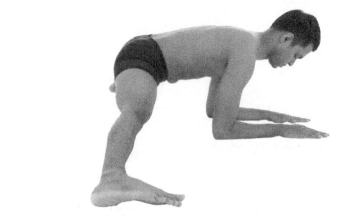

Figure: 183

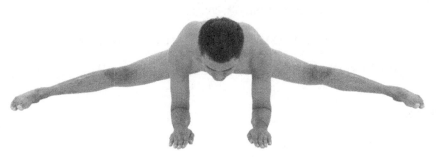

Figure: 184

Step 2:

Gently spread your legs further apart until you can place your elbows on the floor (Figures: 183 and 184). Stay for six breaths.

Advance variation 1:

Stretch you legs wider until you can press your pelvis to the floor. Lay your chest on the floor, stretch your arms out to the sides, and place your palms on the floor (Figure: 185).

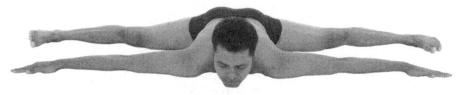

Figure: 185

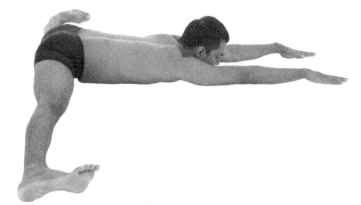

Figure: 186

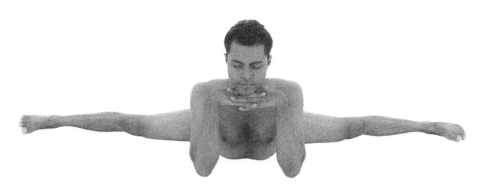

Figure: 187

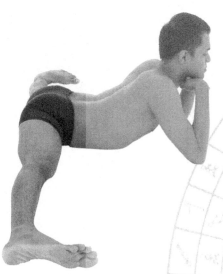

Figure: 188

Advance variation 2:

Once your legs are fully spread out to a 180 degree angle, bring your arms forward (Figure: 186). Then gently arch your spine by pressing your solar plexus on the floor, raise your chest up, and bend your elbows. Interlace your fingers and put your hands under your chin with your palms facing down (Figures: 187 and 188).

191

Pada Anuprasthasana:

Pada: leg, anuprastha: cross. Twisted cross leg pose.

How to enter:

After releasing from samakonasana, place your feet about three feet apart, palms on the floor (Figure: 189). As you exhale, pivot your feet as you turn your torso 180 degrees to the left. Your left leg will be crossing in front of your right leg, keep your feet parallel with each other and pointing straight ahead (Figure: 190). You will be facing the direction on the mat representing West. Keep your knees straight and hips in a neutral position. This asana stretches your hamstrings, outer hips, and buttocks as a compensation for samakonasna. Stay in the pose for six breaths.

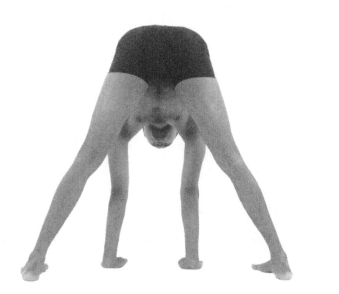

Figure: 189

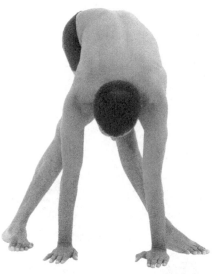

Figure: 190

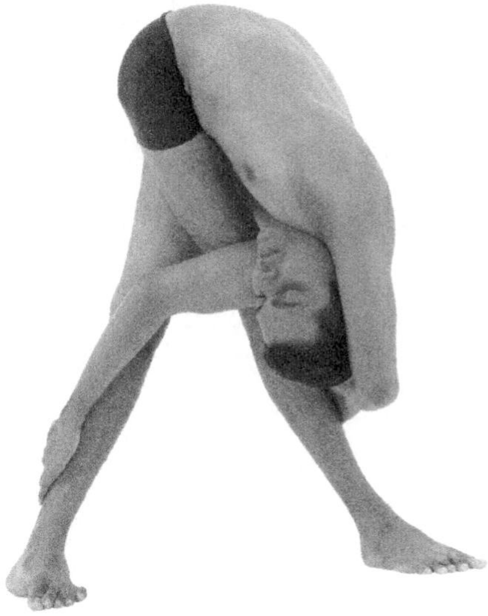

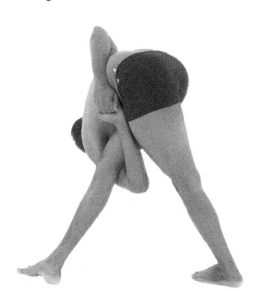

Figure: 191

Advance variation 1:

This variation takes the twist an extra step. If your spine is able to rotate into deep twists, then add this variation. Follow the steps mentioned for the beginning version (Figure: 190). Now use your left hand to grab your left ankle and your right hand to grab your right ankle. Twist your torso and head to the left (Figure: 191).

Figure: 192

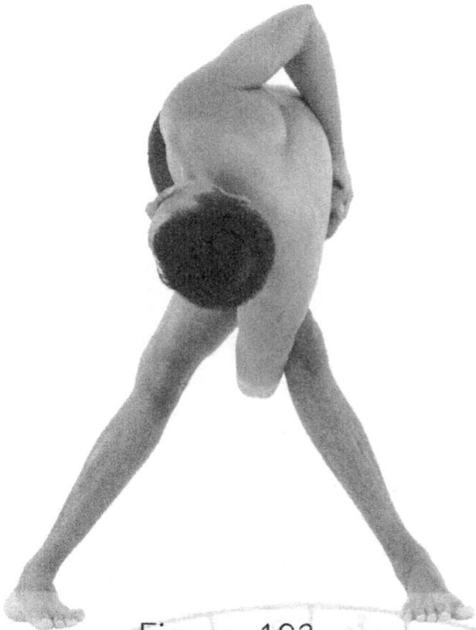

Figure: 193

Advance variation 2:

Follow the steps mentioned for the beginning version (Figure: 190). Then bend your elbows bringing your right arm under your left leg, your left hand behind your back to grab your right hand, and twist your torso deeply (Figures: 192 and 193).

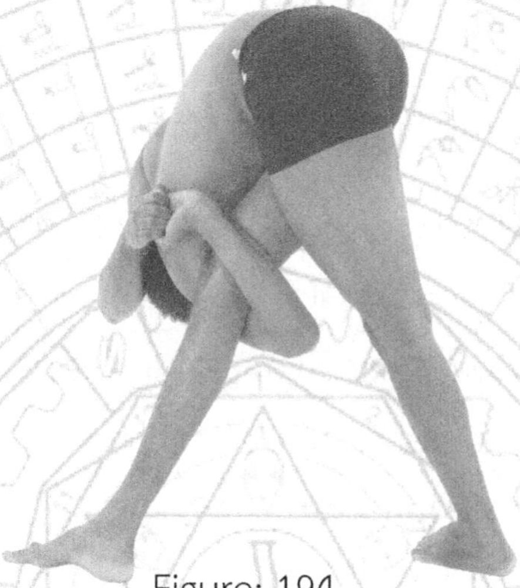

Figure: 194

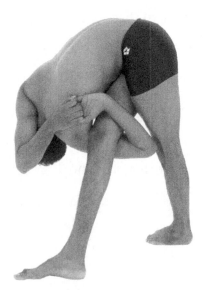

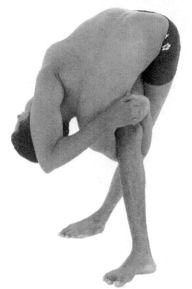

Figure: 195   Figure: 196

Advance variation 3:

This variation binds the hands in gomuka arms. Follow the steps mentioned for the beginning version (Figure: 190). Then bend your right elbow, bring your right arm under your left leg, and put your arm behind your back. Now raise your left arm over your head, bend your elbow, and bind with your right hand (Figures: 194, 195, and 196). Your shoulders will be deeply active, along with having a strong spinal twist. Avoid holding your breath or breathing rapidly. Do not attempt these asanas until you have mastered the easier variations. Practice can help you gradually progress. It is a way to unleash your own potential through regular commitments.

Mirror reflection to your right side:

As you exhale, turn back to your right 180 degrees to the starting position and repeat samakonasana (Figures: 178 - 184). Then release and repeat pada anuprathasthasana to the right side (Figures: 185 - 192). Hold for six breaths, then release.

Vinyasa:

Vinyasa Abdominal Down:

Release from pada anuprasthasana, step back to plank pose. Do one vinyasa abdominal down (Figures: 9, 10 and 11).

From adho mukha svanansa (Figure: 11) shift forward into plank and lower down to lay on the floor.

Orientation:

Face the direction on the mat representing East.

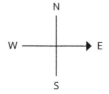

Asanas:

Dwi Bhuja Swastikasana:

Dwi: two; bhuja: arm; swastika: symbol of the swastika. The pose represents the symbol of swastika with two sides of arm variation, hence the name of the pose.

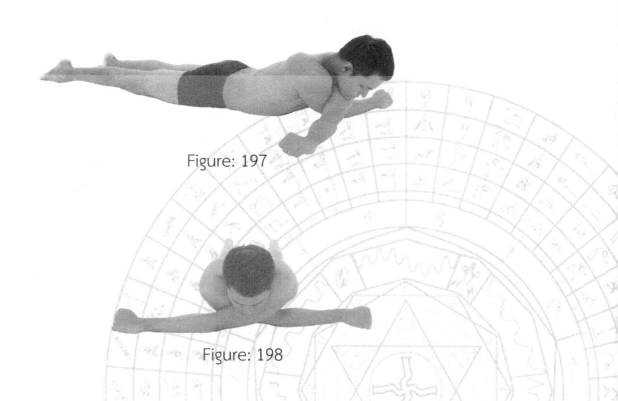

Figure: 197

Figure: 198

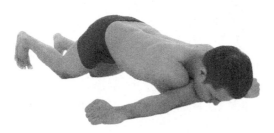

Figure: 199

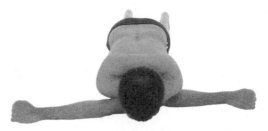

Figure: 200

How to enter:

Lay on your stomach keeping your feet hip width apart. Cross your left arm under the throat, keep the elbow straight, then cross your right arm over your left arm with your palms facing down in mushti mudra (Figures: 197 and 198).

Advance variation 1:

Follow the instructions for the first step (Figure: 197). Then tuck your toes under, bend your knees, and press them into the floor. Lift your hips and chest (Figure: 199). Now move your chest slightly forward to bring your chest over your arms (Figure: 200). If you are feeling like you are crushing your throat, adjust your position to avoid choking the throat or coughing during this pose. If you get numbness or have difficulty with the arms, place a block under the chest and rest on it. This pose gives a deep stretch to the back of the shoulders.

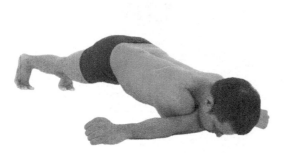

Figure: 201

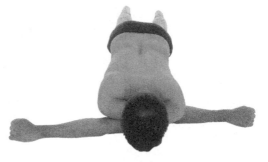

Figure: 202

Advance variation 2:

Apply the same principles from advance variation 1 (Figure: 199). Then press your toes firmly on the floor lifting your knees up (Figure: 201 and 202).

Go directly to baddha dwi bhuja swastikasana before releasing the arms.

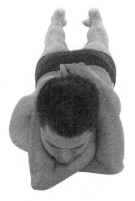

Figure: 203

Baddha Dwi Bhuja Swastikasana:

Baddha: bound; dwi: two; bhuja: arm; swastikasawa: symbol of swastika

Right from dwi bhuja swastikasana, simply bind your hands behind your neck (Figure: 203). Hold for six breaths. As you exhale, release the bind.

Mirror reflection:

Now with the opposite arm on top, repeat dwi bhuja swastikasana and baddha dwi bhuja swastikasana.

Vinyasa:

Vinyasa Abdominal Down:

Release from baddha dwi bhuja swastikasana, step back to plank pose. Do one vinyasa abdominal down (Figures: 9, 10 and 11).

From adho mukha svanansa (Figure: 11) shift forward into plank and lower down to lay on the floor.

Orientation:

Face the direction on the mat representing East.

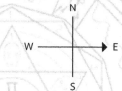

197

Asanas:

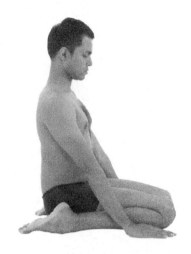

Figure: 204

Supta Virasana:

Supta: lying; vira: brave person, hero

How to enter:

Step 1:

Bend your knees and sit in between your feet. Keep your toes pointing back in plantar flexion. Keep your back erect and place your palms on the floor (Figure: 204).

Step 2:

Exhale and lower your back to the floor. Make sure your knees feel safe by rotating your femur bones internally in the hip sockets. Gradually bring your knees together, bring your hands over your head and elongate your spine. There will be a natural arch to the lower back (Figure: 205).

This asana demands lots of internal rotation at your hips, and it impacts your hip flexors and quadriceps. Your legs are deeply active. Stay in the pose for six breaths.

When you are ready to come upright, inhale, then use momentum, the strength of your abdomen, and your arms sweeping forward to lift your torso up without using your hands for support.

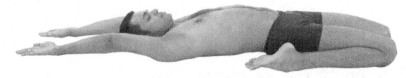

Figure: 205

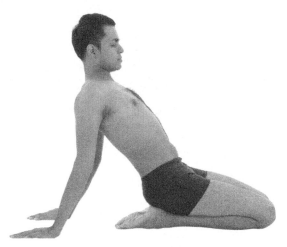

Figure: 206

Modification 1:

If you cannot sit between your feet in supta virasana, practice this modification instead. First bend your knees and sit on your heels. In the beginning, sit straight for couple of breaths. Then as you exhale, lean back and place your palms on the floor behind your back. Keep your head straight and support with your arms (Figure: 206). If it is too hard to place your hands on the floor, use your fingertips.

Beginners can hold this pose for six breaths. As you progress, you could sit in this position for one or two minutes. This pose creates a good beginning stretch. Once you can sit without any trouble, eventually you will be able to try the full expression of the pose by sitting between your feet, then laying back (Figure: 205). If you feel this modification is too hard or causes pain in the knees, then sit on a block.

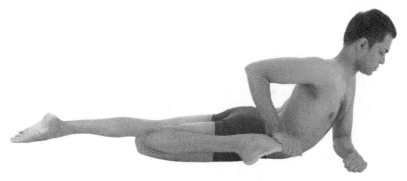

Figure: 207

Bhekasana:

Bheka: frog

How to enter:

After exiting from supta virasana, cross your ankles, roll over your shins, and step back to lie on your stomach. Start with your legs straight, bend your right elbow in front of your chest, and place the forearm in a horizontal position. Now bend your left knee, move it slightly away from the line of your right hip. Now place your left hand on top of your left foot, spin your fingers forward so your toes and fingers point in the same direction (Figure: 207). In order to press the toes and heel down, broaden and rotate your shoulder forward. Your palm works as a lever to push your left toes towards the floor. This creates a deep internal rotation of your left hip. Keep your neck relaxed. Do not aggravate or create any pain around your knees. Keep your right leg straight and active. Hold for six to eight breaths.

Mirror reflection:

Repeat the pose with the opposite knee bent.

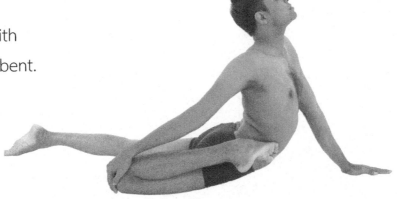

Figure: 208

Advance variation 1:

If you are quite flexible at the knee and hip you can add on from the previous position (Figure: 207). Start by locking your left toes under the left side of your ribcage. Grab your left knee with your left hand, keep your right arm straight in a diagonal line with the palm facing down. Avoid leaning into the shoulder and lift your chest to avoid compression in your lower back. Now arch gently with the support of your left hand (Figure: 208). Hold for six breaths.

Mirror reflection:

Repeat the pose with the opposite knee bent.

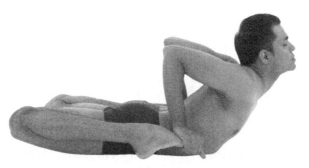

Figure: 209

Advance variation 2:

This is an advance variation of frog pose. Lay on your stomach, bend your knees, and move them slightly away from the line of your hips. Place your hands on top of your feet, spin your fingers forward pointing your toes and fingers in a same direction. As you exhale, lift your head up, simultaneously press the top of your feet down to press the heels and toes towards the floor. Avoid turning your toes out. Keep the hips, quadriceps, and ankles active. With your belly on the floor, expand the top of the torso up (Figure: 209). Keep your eyes closed and steady without any fluctuations in your consciousness. If you encounter any issues around the knees and hips, then practice the modified version of this pose (Figure: 210).

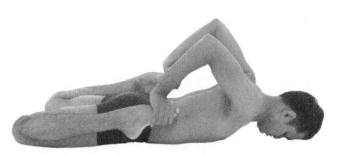

Figure: 210

Modification:

Lay on your stomach, bend your knees, and move them slightly away from the line of your hips. Place your hands on top of your feet, spin your fingers forward pointing your toes and fingers in the same direction. Rest your head on the floor or on a blanket and apply gentle pressure to your feet (Figure: 210).

It is applicable to begin your practice with this modified version before doing the full version of bhekasana (Figure: 209), because you have to prepare your hips, knees, and shoulders. Other simple asanas that use internal rotation of the hips are also beneficial to gain the mobility needed. Through proper practice and dedication you can progress. But if there is sharp pain or aggravation in the knees, then avoid trying to achieve the more advance versions.

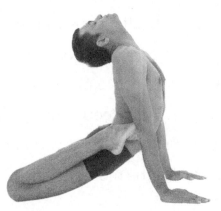

Figure: 211

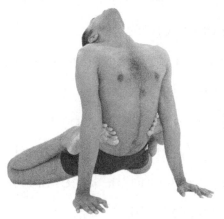

Figure: 212

Advance variation 3:

How to enter:

Lay on your stomach, bend you knees, and slightly move your knees apart. Place your hands on top of your feet, spin your hands as you internally rotate your shoulders forward and hips inward. Toes and fingers point in the same direction. Use the strength of your arms to press your toes firmly on the floor. Lift your chest up off the floor, and slowly pull the knees inward to deeply stretch your quadriceps and hip joints. Now lock your toes under your waist with the support of your hands. Once the toes are locked around your waist, place your hands on the floor in front of your chest. As you inhale, gently arch your back, slowly lift the pubic bone up, looking backward (Figures: 211 and 212). Rest your knees on the floor. Avoid holding your breath. It is not necessary to do this variation every time you practice this sequence. Just play with it once in a while. Stay in the pose for six to eight breaths.

Vinyasa:

Vinyasa Abdominal Down:

After exiting from bhekasana, step back to plank pose. Do one vinyasa abdominal down (Figures: 9, 10 and 11).

Stay in adho mukha svanansa (Figure: 11).

Orientation:

Face the direction on the mat representing East.

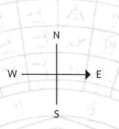

Asanas:

Adho Mukha Svanasana:

Adho: downward; mukha: face, svana: dog

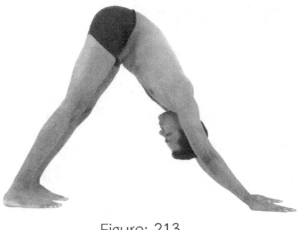

Figure: 213

How to enter:

After the vinyasa abdominal down, you will already be in adho mukha svananasa (Figure: 213). Use this pose to stretch your shoulders, but be sure to keep your shoulder girdle stable and spine long.

Viparitha Namaskarasana:

Viparitha: reverse; namaskar: prayer position. Here the arms are placed in reverse prayer position.

How to enter:

Bend your knees, sit on your heels with toes pointed in plantar flexion. If your knees have any issues then use a prop, like a block or blanket, under your buttocks. As you inhale bend your elbows and spiral your hands behind your back in reverse prayer position. Your shoulders will be internally rotated with palms together. Slightly pull your elbows backward to avoid pressure on your wrists and to help rotate your shoulders deeply inward (Figure: 214).

As you exhale, bend forward and rest your forehead on the floor (Figure: 215). Keep your elbows lifted and gently lengthen your spine. Avoid lifting your buttocks off your heels. Stay for six long breaths. Inhale and come up, then release the arms.

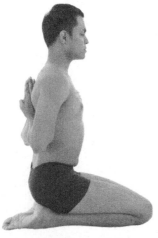

Figure: 214

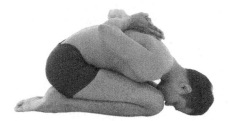

Figure: 215

Vinyasa:

Chakra Vinyasa - Somersault Forward:

Tuck your toes under, place your palms on the floor, and flex your neck bringing your chin toward your chest (Figure: 133). As you exhale, bend forward and place the back of your head onto the floor. As you round your neck further to the floor, gently raise your hips in the air (Figure: 134). Remember to keep your neck relaxed. Now using the strength from your legs and arms, roll forward. Place your upper back on the floor (Figure: 135), then roll forward and sit (Figure: 136).

Orientation:

Face the direction on the mat representing East.

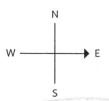

Asanas:

Baddha Konasana:

Baddha: bound; kona: angle. This pose is called bound angle pose, often referred to as cobbler pose.

How to enter:

Sitting on the floor, bend your knees and bring the bottom of your feet together.

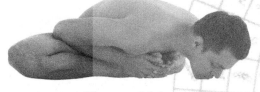

Your hips will be abducted and externally rotated. Bring your heels close to your perineum and interlace your fingers under

Figure: 216

205

your feet. Place your elbows on top of your thighs. Inhale and gradually press your knees down towards the floor. As you exhale, fold your torso forward while lengthening your spine. Once your chin can rest on the floor, you can stretch your arms forward, but still anchor your hips down. It is easy to focus on the front of the body. This will help bring awareness to the back of the body. Keeping your chin on the floor, simultaneously press your sit bones down. This can help to keep you engaged so you don't collapse while statically holding the asana (Figure: 216). Once you can do this pose effortlessly, then hold for six breaths. As you inhale, raise your torso up and release.

Modification:

Bring your feet together, externally rotate your hip joints, and pull your heels back towards your perineum. Gently press your legs down with your elbows. Depending on your flexibility, if the adductors are tight don't push hard as it can lead to knee injury. Gradually access your hip mobility through regular practice. Once your legs lower enough to rest on the floor, lengthen your spine and gently bend forward to get a deeper stretch in your hips and adductors

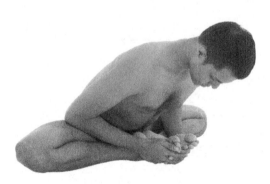

Figure: 217

(Figure: 217). This variation is a great pose for beginners to start with to avoid injuries around the hips.

Note:

During the initial state of my practice, I placed sand bags on my thighs to give gentle pressure on my hips. If you have a person apply pressure for you, be careful that it is gentle. If a partner gives one hundred percentage of their weight to your hips, it can put your hips at risk of a serious injury that could last a lifetime. Therefore, practice cautiously, and ideally with an experienced Universal Yoga teacher. Often with help, you can get results quicker to attain the pose effortlessly.

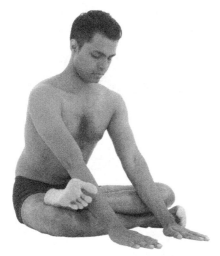

Figure: 218

Dwi Pada Kapotasana:

Dwi: two; pada: leg; kapota: pigeon. This is similar to the one leg pigeon pose variation, but with two legs.

How to enter:

Step 1:

Sitting on the floor with bent knees, externally rotate your right hip and place your right leg on the floor with the knee bent 90 degrees. Then place your left ankle on top of your right knee, keeping your shin bones in a straight line. Dorsiflex your ankles, which helps to keep the knees safe. Place your palms on the floor in front of your shin bones and lengthen your spine (Figure: 218). If your feel intense pain in the hips or any pressure around your knees, back off until you feel more comfortable.

Step 2:

When you are ready to add on, fold your torso forward and gently stretch your arms straight ahead. This will boost the stretch particularly in your glutues medius and minimus. For some people it also affects the gluteus maximus. If your are able to lengthen your spine further, then place your chin on the floor, anchor your your hips down (Figure: 219), and stay for six breaths before releasing.

Modification 1:

This variation is for practitioners with stiff hips. Begin with one leg at a time, rather then starting with both legs. Keep your right leg straight, bend your left

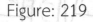

Figure: 219

knee 90 degrees, catch your left ankle with your right hand, and grab your left knee with your left hand (Figure: 220). Place your left ankle on top of your right knee and gently press your left knee down. Keep your left ankle dorsiflexed and hold it firmly (Figure: 221).

This modification is a great start for beginners. Spend time working in this pose during the beginning stage of your practice.

Modification 2:

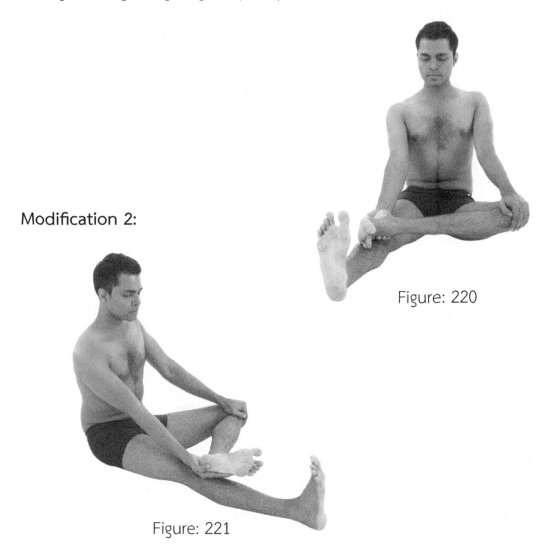

Figure: 220

Figure: 221

Once you are able to perform the first modification easily (Figure: 221), proceed to the first step of double pigeon pose (Figure: 218). In the beginning when the hips are tight, bending the torso forward can create pressure around the knees, hips, and glutues. Therefore, put your palms on the ground behind you, keep

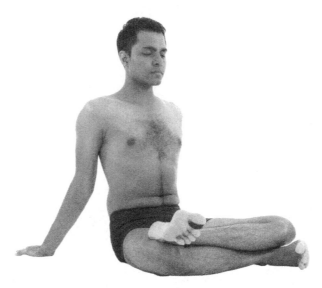

Figure: 222

your back straight and lean back into your hands. Avoid rounding your back. Dorsiflex your ankles to avoid any knee injuries (Figure: 222). If you encounter any acute pain or discomfort, then return back to the previous modified version and continue to practice gradually over a period of time. Once you have progressed enough to do this pose well, then you can try to bend forward to the full version of dwi pada vakrasana (Figure: 219).

Mirror reflection:

Repeat the same variation you did on the first side but now with the right leg on top.

Vinyasa:

Vinyasa Abdomen Up:

Beginner variation 1:

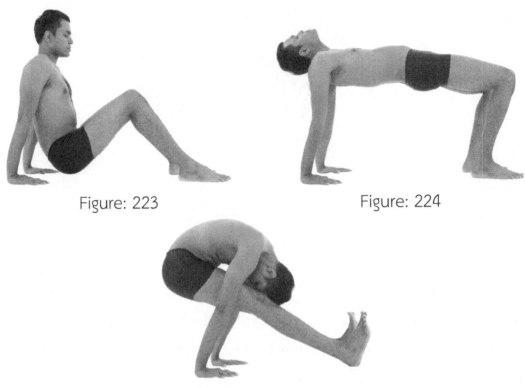

Figure: 223

Figure: 224

Figure: 225

Step 1:

From a seated position, bend your knees, put your feet flat on the floor, and place your hands behind your back with your fingers facing forward (Figure: 223).

Step 2:

As you inhale, lift your hips up and contract your back and gluteus maximus (Figure: 224).

Step 3:

As you exhale, pull your hips back, contract your abdomen muscles, and press your heels down. Your hips will pass through your arms and lift towards the line of your shoulders (Figure: 225). Keep your knees straight and avoid tension in your neck. Feel the natural pause when you pull through on each exhale.

Repeat this vinyasa four times (Figures: 224 and 225).

Beginner variation 2:

This version of vinyasa abdomen up is recommended for beginners to practice to help strengthen the upper body and abdomen muscles. In order to achieve the vinyasa abdomen up effortlessly, you must master the easier variations. Then you can work to attain the full version of this vinyasa.

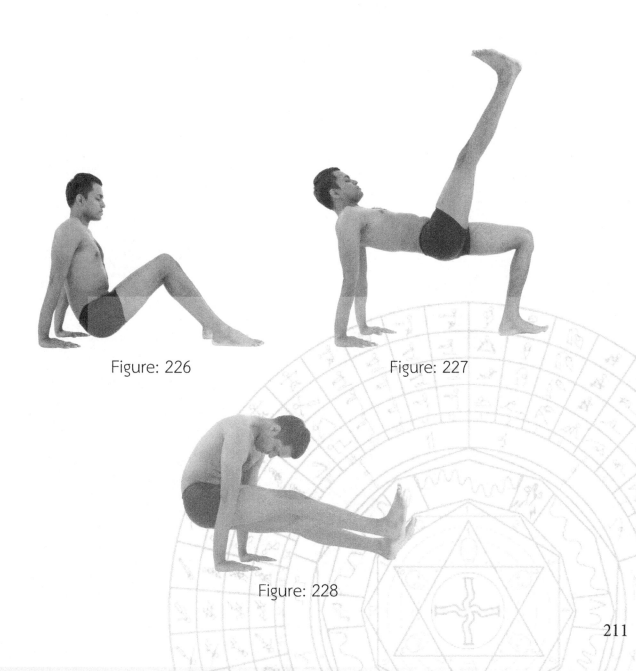

Figure: 226

Figure: 227

Figure: 228

Start the same way as in step one (Figure: 226). Now inhale lifting your hips up and raising your left leg up 90 degrees (Figure: 227). As you exhale, pull your hips back, contract your abdomen muscles, and press your right heel firmly on the ground. Keep your right knee straight and avoid flopping your right foot out to the side. Your hips have to pass through your arms. When you lift the left leg, your left foot will be 20 degrees off the floor (Figure: 228). As you firm your abdomen, you will be able to lift your hips a few inches off the floor with both knees straight. Avoid tension around your neck and wrists. As you inhale again, switch legs and lift your hips up (Figure: 227). Exhale and pull your hips through your arms again (Figure: 228). This completes one round. You can repeat this method for two rounds.

Beginner variation 3:

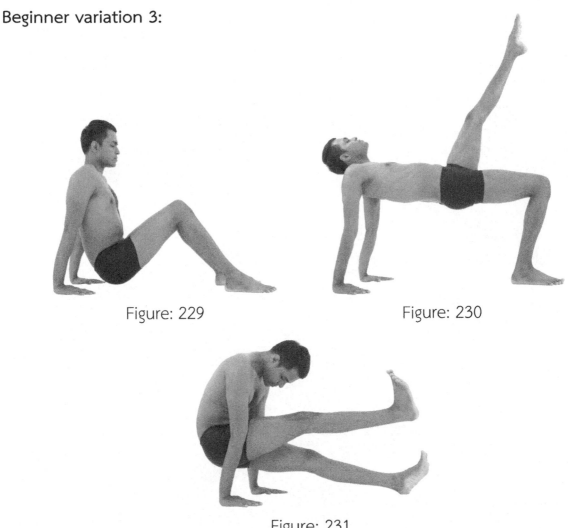

Figure: 229   Figure: 230

Figure: 231

Start with the same principles as you did for the second beginner variation (Figures: 229 and 230). Except as you exhale, pull your hips back and lift your right leg higher to a 45 degree angle (Figure: 231). As a result, your right foot will go above your shoulders and head. If you have practiced the previous variations faithfully, then this variation will not be as hard to attain. Regular practice can bring the fruits of success.

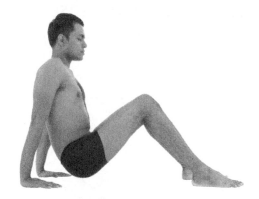

Figure: 232

Advance variation:

This variation demands a lot of strength in the arms, abdomen, and legs. It is not advised for beginners to perform. Once you can do the beginner vinyasa abdomen up variations fairly easy, then you can start applying this method without as much difficulty.

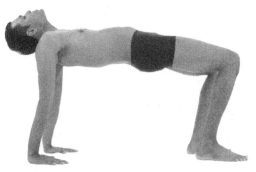

Figure: 233

As you inhale lift your hips up (Figure: 233) and as you exhale pull your hips backwards between your arms and lift your legs high on the air (Figure: 234). Repeat a total of four times. Then place your feet back on the floor and lift your pelvis (Figure: 233) to complete the vinyasa. Then sit on the floor.

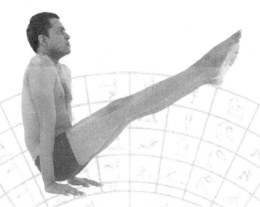

Figure: 234

Orientation:

Face the direction on the mat representing East.

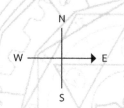

213

Asanas:

Eka Bhuja Kapotasana 6:

Eka: one; bhuja: arm; kapota: pigeon. Another variation of kapotasana for the arms.

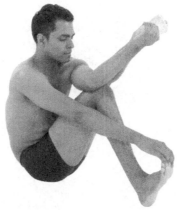

Figure: 235

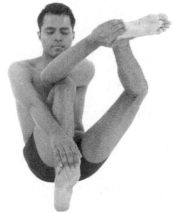

Figure: 236

How to enter:

Sit on the floor with knees bent facing up. As you inhale, lift your left leg and hold the outer heel with your left palm. Keep your wrist neutral, to avoid extending it backward. Place the left outer elbow on the right outer edge of your knee. Keep your left forearm at a diagonal with the elbow bent 90 degrees. As you exhale, press your left leg down as a lever to externally rotate your left

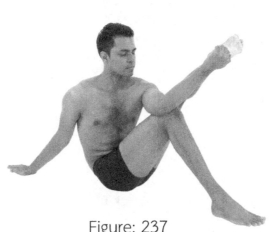

Figure: 237

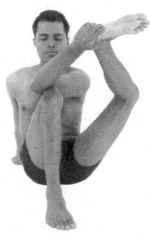

Figure: 238

shoulder. Adjust the pressure according to your shoulder mobility. Now catch the ball of your right foot with your right hand and press the right toes forward to get a deeper shoulder stretch (Figures: 235 and 236).

Modification 1:

If your shoulders are tight, then place your right hand on the floor behind the line of your right sit bone (Figures: 237 and 238), to provide support to stretch your left shoulder and elbow. Keep your back erect and your hips in a neutral position.

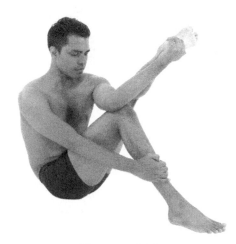

Figure: 239

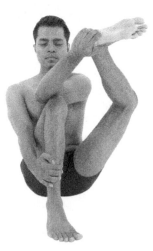

Figure: 240

Modification 2:

Apply the same principle as described in the first modification (Figure: 237). If your shoulder mobility is getting more effortless, then lengthen your spine and bring your right hand forward to grab your right shin (Figures: 239 and 240). Avoid moving your right leg out. Hold for six long breaths, then release.

Eka Bhuja Kapotasana 4:

Another variation of kapotasana for the arms, but with an internal rotation of the shoulder.

This is a counter stretch to the previous eka bhuja kapotasana. Therefore continue working with the first arm, then you will change sides and repeat both poses.

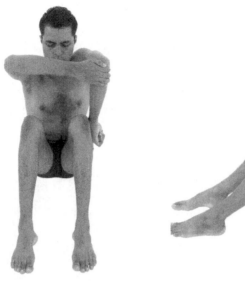

Figure: 242

Figure: 241

How to enter:

Sit on the floor, bend your knees keeping them hip distance apart with your feet flat on the floor. Turn your left shoulder inward and place the back of your left wrist on the outer edge of your left knee. Grab your left arm from below the line of your elbow. As you exhale, pull your left shoulder inward so both shoulders are in a straight line. When you look from above, the arms will look like a square. Keep your legs strong so you can press your left wrist firmly against the left outer knee without moving the leg. Lengthen your spine, keep your head in the line of the spine (Figures: 241 and 242). Stay for six long breaths. Then inhale and release from the shoulder stretch.

Mirror reflection:

Once you finish eka bhuja kapotasana 6 and eka bhuja kapotasana 4 with the left arm consecutively, then repeat using the right arm.

Vinyasa:

Vinyasa Abdomen Up:

From a sitting position, bend your knees with your feet flat on the floor. Put your hands behind your back with your fingers facing forward (Figure: 223). Choose the version of vinyasa abdominal up that you are capable of executing. Repeat this vinyasa four times (Figures: 224 and 225; 227 and 228; 230 and 231; or 233 and 234).

Orientation:

Face the direction on the mat representing East.

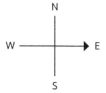

Asanas:

Baddha Padma Navasana:

Baddha: bound; padma: lotus; navasana: resembles the shape of a boat.

How to enter:

Baddha padma navasana is one of the great balancing poses. In order to do this pose, you must have experience practicing simple balancing positions on your sit bones. Without experience, sitting in lotus position can cause tension around your ankles and knees. This pose uses external rotation of your hips, if they are stiff, then it's better to initiate practice with one of the modifications.

Step 1:

Sit on the floor with straight legs, then bend your left knee, and place your left foot on top of the right edge of your thigh. Bend your right knee and place your right foot on top of the left edge of your thigh in lotus position. Now place your hands on the outside

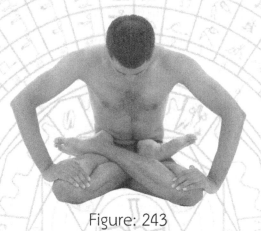

Figure: 243

of your knees and gently squeeze your knees in (Figure: 243). This can help you become fixed in the pose. Avoid pressure around the knees.

Step 2 :

Keep your spine straight, place your hands on the outer edge of your knees, and inhale while lifting your knees up. The soles of your feet will be resting at the bottom of your ribcage and you will be balancing on your sit bones. Avoid collapsing back onto your tailbone. Now wrap your arms around the outside of your legs. If the spine is long then gently clasp your fingers (Figure: 244).

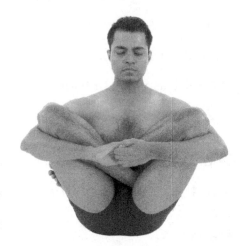

Figure: 244

Step 3:

If you have got enough flexibility, then catch your wrist firmly (Figure: 245). Avoid falling backward and hold for six breaths.

Modification 1:

Ardha Padmasana:

Ardha: half; padma: lotus.

There are different stages to modifications. All of the variations are necessary to progress.

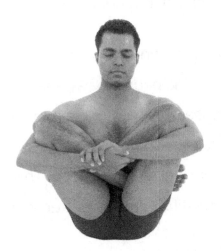

Figure: 245

Choose your modification according to your physical condition. Doing the final stage of this pose without warm up on your legs can put pressure on your knees. Therefore, you can begin practicing with one leg.

Sit on the floor with both legs straight. Now bend your left knee and place your left foot on top of the right edge of your upper thigh. If you feel any discomfort

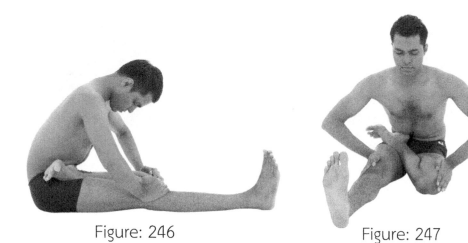

Figure: 246

Figure: 247

attempting this first stage, then place a block or rolled towel under your knee. This can help you access the mobility in your hips gradually, taking the pressure off your knees. Once you place your leg in half lotus pose, then gently squeeze your legs in (Figures: 246 and 247). Don't push too strong on your knees. Once in the pose, hold for six breaths.

Modification 2:

Apply the same principles mentioned in the first modification (Figure: 246). Now fold your torso forward, catching the heel of your foot with your hands. Rest your right shoulder on top of your right knee. Rest your head on the floor (Figure: 248 and 249).

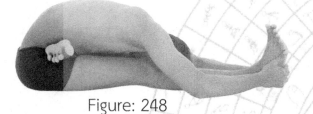

Figure: 248

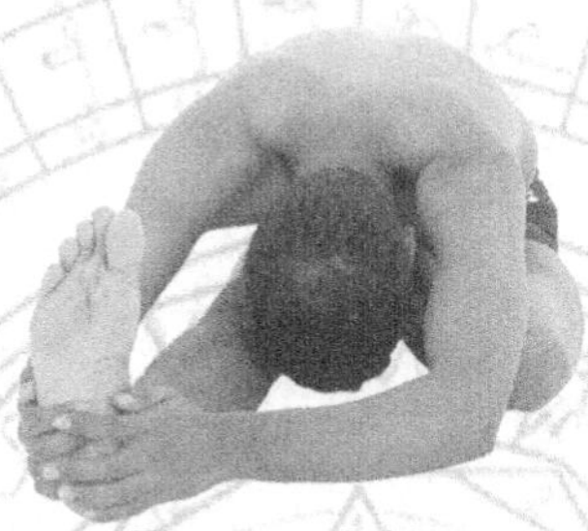

Figure: 249

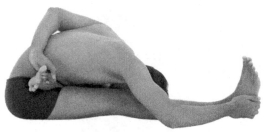

Figure: 250

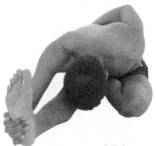

Figure: 251

Modification 3:

Ardha Baddha Padmasana:

Ardha: half; baddha: bound; padma: lotus.

Follow the same principles mentioned in the second modification. Then bend your left elbow and bring your left arm behind your back to grab your left foot. Fold forward catching your right heel with your right hand. As you lengthen your spine, rest your right shoulder on top of your right knee. Keep your hips and spine even. Stretch your hamstrings deeply (Figure: 250 and 251).

Advance variation 1:

Baddha Padmasana:

Baddha: bound; padma: lotus.

If you are able to perform baddha padma navasana (Figure: 245) well while staying relaxed, then try this variation. An important element of flexibility for this pose, besides in the hips, is in the shoulders. Tight shoulders can cause difficulty reaching the big toes. Be sure you have cultivated hip, knee, and shoulder flexibility before trying this pose.

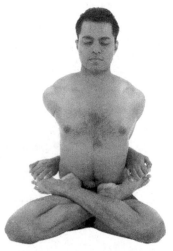

Figure: 252

From lotus position, cross your arms behind your back and catch your toes (Figure: 252). Avoid leaning to one side. Keep your knees grounded. In the beginning, this pose could put pressure on your outer shins and ankles. As you progress, the discomfort subsides.

Advance variation 2:

Follow the directions for the first advance variation (Figure: 252). Once you have grabbed both sides of your feet firmly, press your knees down on the floor and bend your torso forward. Exhale while bringing your chin down to the floor (Figure: 253 and 254).

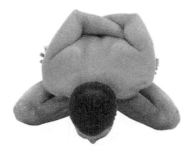

Figure: 253

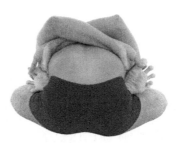

Figure: 254

Note:

Practicing lotus pose itself can be quite intense for the hips, knees, and ankles. In order to take pressure off your knees and hips, you have to cultivate a certain amount of flexibility around your gluteus maximus and medius. Then you can move on to your hips; you have to actively work towards increasing the external rotation of your hips. Practice poses such as dwi pada vakrasana, baddha konasana, etc. Then lotus will slowly become accessible and comfortable. Also work with your shoulders. In order to bind your hands to your feet behind your back, you must have good medial rotation of your shoulders. Stiff shoulders can restrict doing the end stage of baddha padmasana. Therefore, practice the shoulder poses regularly to stretch your deltoids, pectoralis major and minor, trapezius, and the posterior part of the shoulders. Please remember that over practicing can lead to injury around your shoulders. They are delicate to stretch. Know your limitations, progress gradually, and with patience.

Mirror reflection:
Repeat the pose variation you choose using the opposite side.

Vinyasa:

Vinyasa Abdomen Up:
Release from baddha padma navasana. Bend your knees with your feet flat on the floor. Put your hands behind your back with your fingers facing forward (Figure: 223). Choose the version of vinyasa abdominal up that you are capable of executing. Repeat this vinyasa four times (Figures: 224 and 225; 227 and 228; 230 and 231; or 233 and 234).

Orientation:
Face the direction on the mat representing East.

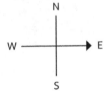

Asanas:

Bhuja Paripurna Virasana:
Bhuja: arms; paripurna: complete version of posture; vira: hero. This pose re-sembles a complete internal rotation of the shoulder.

How to enter:
Sit on the floor with your knees bent and your feet flat on the floor. As you inhale, bend your elbows and place the back of your palms and wrists on your outer side of your ribcage. Keep your fingers locked in mushti mudra. Bring your elbows to the inside of your knees. As you exhale, squeeze your knees in to apply a stretch on your shoulders (Figure: 255). Do not let your wrists slide

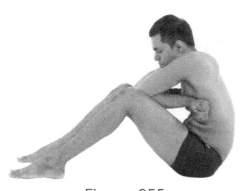

Figure: 255

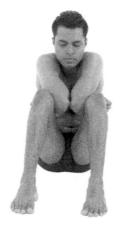

Figure: 256

toward the front part of your ribcage while your knees are squeezing in. This is a deep internal rotation shoulder stretch. As you stretch, move your elbows closer to each other (Figure: 256). Hold for six breaths. Feel the shoulder sensations right after your release from the pose.

This asana works on the deltoids, latissmus dorsi, rhomboids, and elbows. It's an overall package for your shoulders and elbows. To create as deep of a stretch as possible, choose the pose wisely. It's not a main concern to copy the pose exactly as it was shown. If your shoulder flexibility is limited, avoid getting into the final pose immediately. Feel the sensations from the inside, be here and now with a sense of detachment from your body and mind.

Modification 1:

This modified version is suitable for beginners working towards shoulder flexibility. Try to catch your elbows inside your knees like it was described in the first option, except start with feet and knees wider. The main focus in the version, rather then squeezing the knees in, keep the knees apart and hold for couple of breaths without any pressure from outside (Figures: 257 and 258).

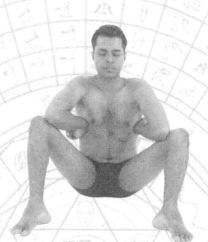

Figure: 257

223

If your shoulders are very tight and its painful to do the pose or you can't get both arms inside the knees, then apply the same principle using one arm at a time. Once you finish one side then change to the opposite side. When it becomes easy with a single arm, then go back to trying it with both arms (Figure: 258). Practicing this modification will help you achieve the full variation eventually.

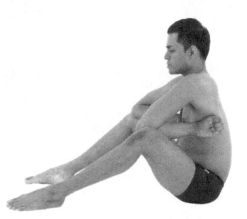

Figure: 258

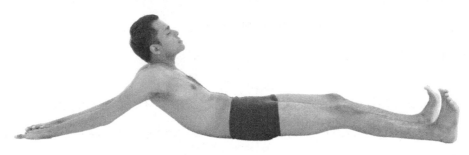

Figure: 259

Nidhanikasana:

Nidhanika: rack

How to enter:

Sit on the floor, interlace your fingers behind your back, and stretch your shoulders deeply by rotating them externally. The inside of your elbows will be facing the floor (Figure: 259). Wiggle your pelvis forward until you rest your lower back on the floor. Have a sense of lifting the chest up so your spine will not be rounded and hunched. While you stretch your legs forward, press your heels on the floor, and bend your knees slightly. Pull with your heels and expand your chest up (Figure: 260). In this lateral rotation shoulder stretch, you will stretch your pectoralis major, anterior deltoids, and your arms. Get the maximum stretch possible. Stay for six long breaths and then release.

Modification 1:

In this modified variation, place your hands behind your buttocks, palms facing down and fingers back. Keep your arms straight and in line with your shoulders (Figure: 261).

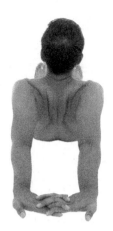

Figure: 260

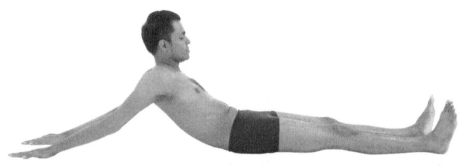

Figure: 261

As you inhale, bend your knees, feet flat on the floor, and lift your buttocks up to move your hips further forward. On an exhale, move even further if you can and rest your lower back on the floor. Eventually, lift your chest up and straighten your legs (Figure: 262).

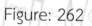

Figure: 262

225

Vinyasa:

Vinyasa Abdomen Up:

Release from nidhanikasana, bend your knees with your feet flat on the floor, and put your hands behind your back with your fingers facing forward (Figure: 223). Choose the version of vinyasa abdominal up that you are capable of executing. Repeat this vinyasa four times (Figures: 224 and 225; 227 and 228; 230 and 231; or 233 and 234).

Orientation:

Face the direction on the mat representing East.

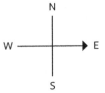

Asanas:

Note:

Chakrasana is listed as Part 1 and setu bandhasana is Part 2 because as you finish chakrasana, you should move directly to setu bandhasana without taking a break. The same procedure should be followed if you are attempting one of the advance variations. There are three options from beginning to very advanced (A, B or C). Choose the variation based on your skill level for this set. Then once you have finished the two consecutive poses, you can relax and lay on your back with your arms overhead.

Chakrasana (Part 1 - Option A):

Chakra: wheel or circular shape. This asana resembles a circle or wheel, hence the name.

How to enter:

Lay on your back, bend your knees, and keep your feet hip distance apart and flat. Extend your arms over your head and bend your elbows. Place your palms under your shoulders and direct your fingers towards you.

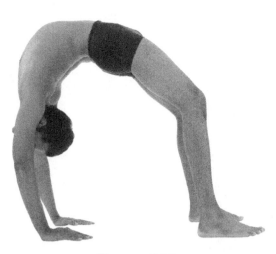

Figure: 263

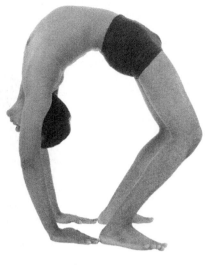

Figure: 264

As you exhale, lift your torso up, keep your elbows straight, and turn your thighs inward which helps to keep your feet in line with your hips (Figure: 263). If the psoas or illiac is stiff, then your feet will tend to open out. If the lower back or shoulders are tight, then it can be hard to keep the arms straight. Therefore, analyze your practice, find the strengths and weaknesses in your body. Then you can make adjustments to correct the imbalances so you perform these advance asanas correctly, rather than pushing hard into the desired postures. Hold for six breaths, then go directly to setu bandhasana (Figure: 266) without taking a break.

Advance variation 1:

Chakra Bandhasana A (Part 1 - Option B):

Chakra is an another form of a yantra representing the psychic energy center, which is a circular shape. Bandha means bound or lock. This pose resembles a full wheel.

This is for advanced students only. If your upper and lower body are very supple, then bring your hands closer to your feet (Figure: 264). From here go directly to vrishchikasana (Figure: 267).

227

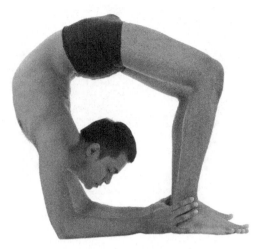

Figure: 265

Advance variation 2:

Chakra Bandhasana B (Part 1 - Option C):

Chakra bandhasana B is quite intense. This is the most incredible backbending asana I have ever found.

To get into this pose, once you have lifted into chakrasana (Figure: 263), bend your elbows and place them on the floor. Keep your body in as deep of an extension as possible, but avoid pushing only through your lower back. Try to activate the muscles of your thoracic spine to extend your back. As you exhale, go deeper into the pose and grab your ankles with your hands. Extend your neck as deeply as you can, do not hold your breath.

In the beginning it may feel like you cannot breath properly. As you progress, the breath starts to settle down and the pressure around the face will start to relax. Hold the pose for six breaths. Then bring your chin to the floor right into vrishchikasana.

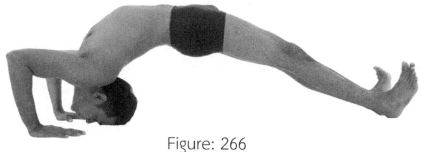

Figure: 266

Setu Bandhasana (Part 2 - Option A):

Setu: bridge; bandha: bound, lock

How to enter:

From chakrasana, bend your elbows, tilt your head back, and place the crown of your head on the floor. If you have cultivated enough neck strength, place your forehead on the floor and straighten your legs. Gradually dorsiflex your feet and press your heels firmly on the ground (Figure: 266).

This pose can put a lot of pressure on your neck so it is important to keep your body symmetrical. The front of your neck extends deeply in this pose. As you practice regularly, start to move your nose towards the floor. Hold for six breaths, then bend your knees, and bring your feet closer so you can lift up and tuck your chin towards your chest to release down to the floor.

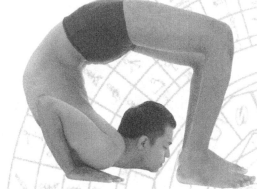

Figure: 267

229

Vrishchikasana (Part 2 - Option B or C):

Vrishchika: scorpion. This is an advance variation of scorpion pose.

How to enter:

From chakra bandhasana A, bend your elbows, tilt your head up and place your chin on the floor (Figure: 267). If you are coming from chakra bandhasana B, lower your chin to the floor while keeping forearms on floor. Hold for six breaths. Release by pushing your palms into the floor and lifting back up. Walk your feet forward a little so you have room to tuck your chin toward your chest and lower your back to the floor.

Bring your arms over your head and straighten your legs. Feel the post effect from the previous poses.

Vinyasa:

Vinyasa Abdomen Up:

Sit up, bend your knees, feet flat on the floor, and put your hands behind your back with your fingers facing forward (Figure: 223). Choose the version of vinyasa abdominal up that you are capable of executing. Repeat this vinyasa four times (Figures: 224 and 225; 227 and 228; 230 and 231; or 233 and 234).

Orientation:

Face the direction on the mat representing East.

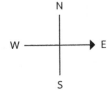

Asanas:

Note:

For the next two poses, you have a choice of practicing Option 1 which includes kurmasana and halasana, or Option 2 which includes yogi nidrasana and maha halasana. You will go directly from one pose into the next just like you did in the previous set.

Kurmasana (Option 1 - Part 1):

Kurma: tortoise. This pose resembles the shape of a tortoise.

How to enter:

Step 1:

Sit on the floor. Inhale and widen your legs. Exhale and bend your knees, folding your torso forward. Now place your arms under your legs and slide them out wide with your palms facing down (Figures: 268 and 269). The bottom of your thighs are now wrapped over the shoulders. If your hamstrings are tight, then hold here.

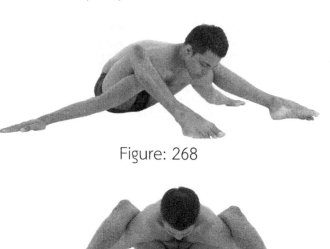

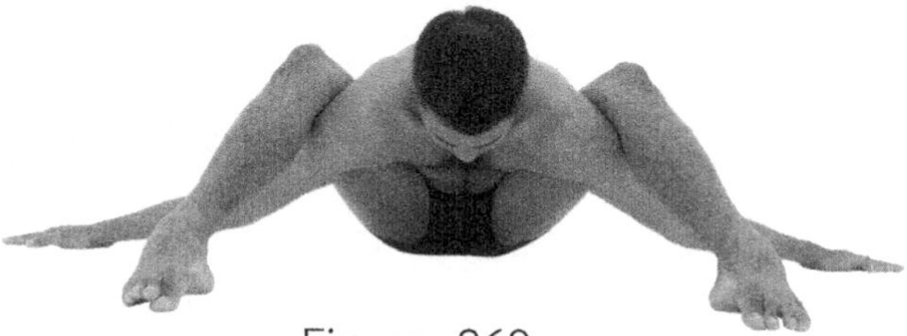

Figure: 268

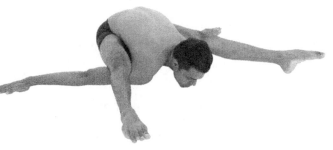

Figure: 269

Step 2:

If your body feels ready, press your feet forward to straighten your legs. Don't spread your

Figure: 270

feet wider, rather push your legs straight ahead. Extend your back to place your chin and solar plexus on the floor (Figure: 270). Bring your hands into mushti mudra (Figure: 271). Hamstring flexibility plays a major role in this pose, along with being able to extend your spine. Hold for six long breaths. After you release roll back directly into the next pose, halasana (Figure: 275).

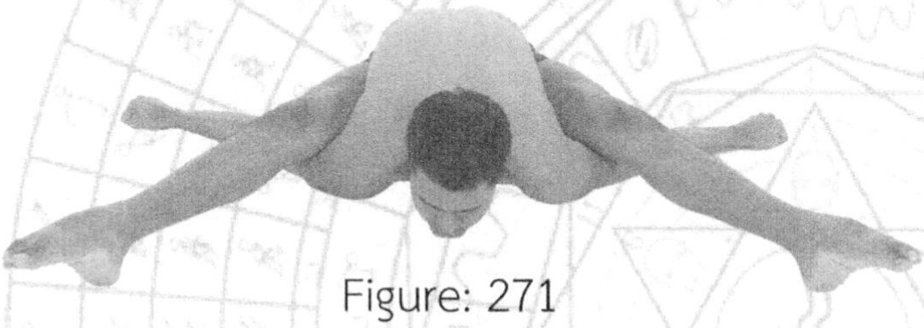

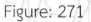

Figure: 271

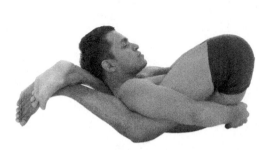

Figure: 272

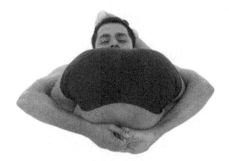

Figure: 273

Yoga Nidrasana (Option 2 - Part 1):

Yoga nidra: conscious sleep. A yogi is relaxed and restful in this stage, yet awake, established, and fully aware.

How to enter:

This is one of the deepest forward bending asanas. It impacts your entire spinal column. Start by laying on your back. As you exhale, bend your knees and bring your left leg behind your arm and around the back of your neck. Move your left shoulders forward to secure your left leg deeply behind your head. Exhale again and bring your right leg behind the back of your neck, hooking it under the left leg firmly. Now nudge your shoulders further through the legs and move your legs deeper under the neck. Bend your elbows, wrap your arms around your legs and behind your back, clasping your fingers (Figure: 272). As you feel the asana becoming easier, hold the grip of the legs firmly, so they will not slide away when you bind your arms. Now push your head up against your legs. As your legs starts moving down, gaze towards the ceiling or close your eyes (Figure: 273). Once you have gotten into the pose, hold it for six long breaths. When you release, go directly to the next pose, maha halasana (Figure: 276).

Halasana (Option 1 - Part 2):

Hala: plow

How to enter:

Step 1:

From kurmasana, sit up and roll onto your back. Bring your feet together and keep your arms

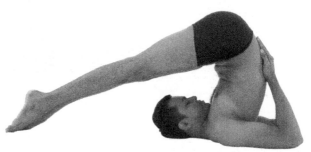

Figure: 274

resting on the floor beside your thighs, with your palms facing down. As you inhale, lift your legs and torso up into a vertical position. Bend your elbows and catch your waist with your palms. You will be supported by your upper arms and head.

Step 2:

As you exhale, gently bring your legs over your head with your toes pointed in plantar flexion (Figure: 274). If it's hard to bring your toes to the floor, hold your legs a few inches off the ground, or place a bolster or block under the feet. Once your toes touch the ground freely, lift your hips higher and lengthen your spine (Figure: 275). Keep your thighs engaged to maintain a good grip on the floor. The neck is in deep flexion. As you gain more access in this pose, your will feel less pressure on your neck. Avoid breathing erratically or holding your breath. In the beginning, you will experience a regular breathing pace. Once you gain control, slow down your breathing and hold the pose for six breaths before releasing.

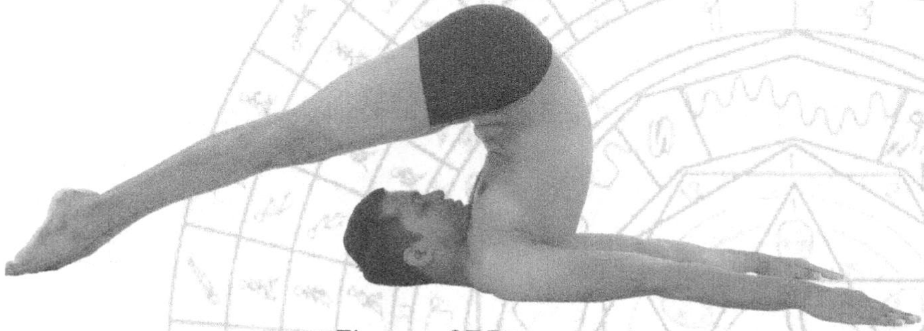

Figure: 275

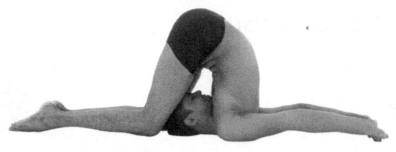

Figure: 276

Maha Halasana (Option 2 - Part 2):

Maha: great; hala: plow. This is the complete variation of halasana.

How to enter:

Apply the same maneuver as mentioned for halasana (Figure: 275). Once hala-sana has become easy from practicing consistently, then bend your knees, keep them together, and gradually bring them to your forehead. In the final stage of this pose, place your knees on the floor over your head and keep your toes pointed. Interlace your fingers and push your palms outward ((Figure: 276). Hold the pose for six deep and relaxing breaths, then go directly to the vinyasa.

Vinyasa:

Ardha Chakra Vinyasa - Half Somersault Backward:

From halasana or maha halasana, place your hands by your head with your fingers pointing towards your shoulders. Roll backwards by pressing your toes on the floor simultaneously pressing your palms firmly under your shoulders, and lifting your hips up over your head (Figure: 161). When you roll back, use momentum and the strength of your hands, legs, and the back of your neck to roll backwards. Then rest your knees on the floor (Figure: 162). Push into your hands to come up (Figure: 163).

Orientation:

Face the direction on the mat representing East.

Asana:

Sirsasana (Option 1):

Sira: head. This pose is called headstand.

Inversions can be fun poses to play around with and master. Practicing inversions can increase arm and upper back strength. But more importantly, you create an energy flow which helps to maintain steady balance and focus on the physical, energetic and spiritual levels.

Ancient people used to dangle down from tree branches, thinking that energy would go towards the head and one could reach the state of kaivalya as a result. However, it is not possible to gain access on the spiritual level by merely dangling upside down; rather a true disciplinary practice is needed. Do not emphasize the asana part alone. When talking about creating a disciplinary practice, you create a sankalpa with what you are doing. A strong sankalpa helps to cultivate the way of looking at your own life. I'm being careful when I say look at 'your own life', because sometimes when you look at yourself, you get caught into finding faults with yourself. You can restrict the body in the actions that you do. Those restrictions can cause tension within you. Just look at your own emotional patterns.

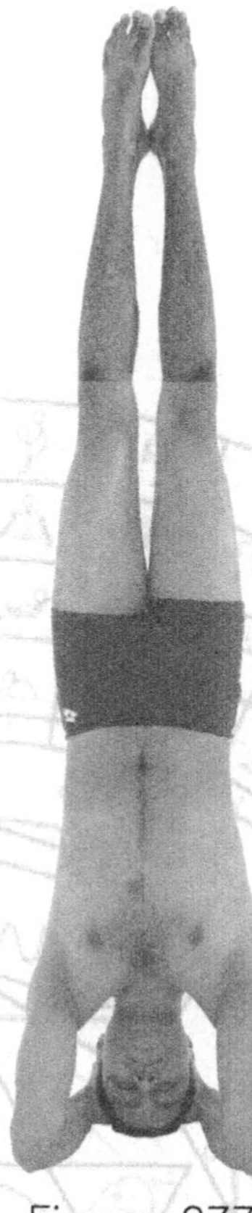

It's good to do inversions to improve your energetic flow, stimulate the glandular actions, or activate the breath. Play with these techniques to see how the results work for you. Some say inversion can help to boost energy, whereas, others says that inversions can help them to sleep better. Be mindful during and after your practice to see how it affects you. Try these asanas out. There are many benefits from inversions. Besides energy moving up, the very effort from

Figure: 277

being willing to learn, and your will can help you alter your state of consciousness to go to the next level.

How to enter:

The myth is that you have to put all of your weight on your neck and head. This is not true. Although you might put all your weight on your head in very advanced versions, in the beginning, there can be little weight on the head and neck. Instead, use your arm and upper body strength, including your deltoids and serrates anterior muscles. This helps to avoid tensing the neck or shrugging the shoulders.

Step 1:

From a kneeling position, place your forearms on the floor with your elbows shoulder distance apart. Interlace your fingers keeping the bottom pinky finger tucked inside your palm, so you will not crush it. Lift your hips up, then place the crown

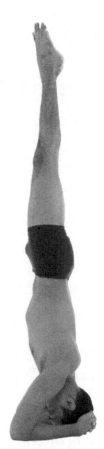

Figure: 278

of your head on the floor. Your palms are against the back of the head. Avoid rounding your neck.

Step 2:

Now press the toes into the floor and walk your feet closer to your face to bring your hips over your head. Make sure your hamstrings are flexible enough, so you don't hunch your back or tilt your pelvis backward.

Step 3:

Now float your legs up so your torso and legs are vertical (Figures: 277 and 278). In the beginning, you can bend your knees and use a lot of core strength to lift up. As you progress, you can keep your legs straight without much effort.

With regular practice, you will feel the weight going to your elbows, forearms, wrists, shoulders, and head. Learn to distribute the weight equally. Breathe long,

236

slow breaths. Don't clench your jaw. Stay for ten breaths, then release the legs slowly to the floor.

Pincha Mayurasana (Option 2):

Pincha: feather; mayura: peacock. Feathered peacock pose also called forearm balance.

How to enter:

From a kneeling position, place your forearms on the floor keeping your elbows in line with your shoulders. Tuck your toes under, lift your hips up and bring one leg up in the air. As you inhale, swing your top leg up as you hop your bottom leg up swiftly (Figure: 279). Avoid falling backwards.

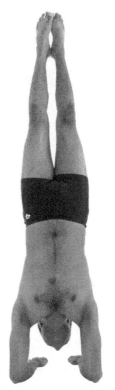

Figure: 279

If you have never tried forearm balance before, practice with a wall behind you for support. If you know how to do it well, then float one leg up at a time without hopping, or hop both legs up at the same time. Keep your legs together, straight, and not wobbling. Keep your legs, hips and head in one line, avoid arching your back. Ensure your big toes are together, contract your belly, and gaze towards the line of your forearm (Figure: 280). Your deltoids, triceps, forearms, serratus anterior, latissimus dorsi, pelvic muscles, back muscles, thighs and legs will all come into play. This understanding alone will not help you achieve the pose, rather regular practice and learning from your own experience will help. Avoid creating tension in your shoulder girdle and neck, tension can create pressure. From the outside, one might look good in the posture,

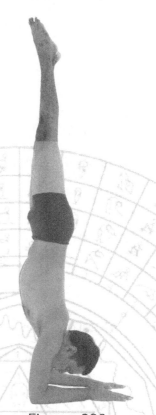

Figure: 280

but what you feel inside matters the most. When you are upside down you can still control the body's capability. You can bring the state of lightness in these inversion postures as well. Hold for six to ten breaths, then release the legs to the floor and rest.

Adho Mukha Vrikshasana (Option 3):

Adho: downward; mukha: face; vriksha: tree. Here you face down with the support of your arms, balancing steady like a tree.

How to enter:

This is an advanced asana. It is best to learn to balance sirsasana (Figure: 278) before you attempt this pose. Overcoming fear is one of the crucial step to learn when you begin your handstand journey. Therefore, initially practice in front of a wall. After you have enough strength in your arms, then you can perform it in the middle of the room without fear.

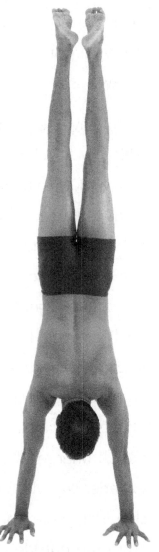

Step 1:

From a kneeling position, place your hands on the floor shoulder width apart, and lift your hips up. Spread your fingers apart to have a good grip on the floor.

Step 2:

Now hop your leg up into vertical position. You will either hop up with one leg or with both legs together, that can change depending on your experience. Once you are vertical, lengthen your spine and avoid arching your lower back (Figure: 281). Keep your belly engaged, bring your big toes together, and find your

Figure: 281

center of gravity in this inverted position. Keep your neck neutral if you can (Figure: 282).

In the beginning it is perfectly fine to tilt your head up. As you progress, your upper body strength comes more into play. Your core muscles, deltoids, serrates anterior, and lattisimus dorsi are all involved to reach this incredible position. If you have your balance, then hold up to ten long breaths. If you are practicing with the support of the wall, then hold from ten to twenty breaths regularly, without falling.

When you are ready to release, don't let gravity pull your legs down so you fall on the floor. Rather come down slowly and with control. Rest in child's pose for a few breaths.

Note:

There are three options for the final inversion in this sequence, headstand (Figure: 278), forearm balance (Figure: 280), and handstand (Figure: 282). These three options have been shown in order of difficulty for your reference, not so you try all three in one practice. Choose one of the inversion poses based on your body's capability. As you progress, choose the handstand variation over the other two options.

Once you have increased your training form, you can use handstand as the vinyasa in place of vinyasa abdominal down and vinyasa side down in the sequence. This will increase the intensity of the practice. Always be aware of your energy during practice so you can keep your endurance throughout the practice.

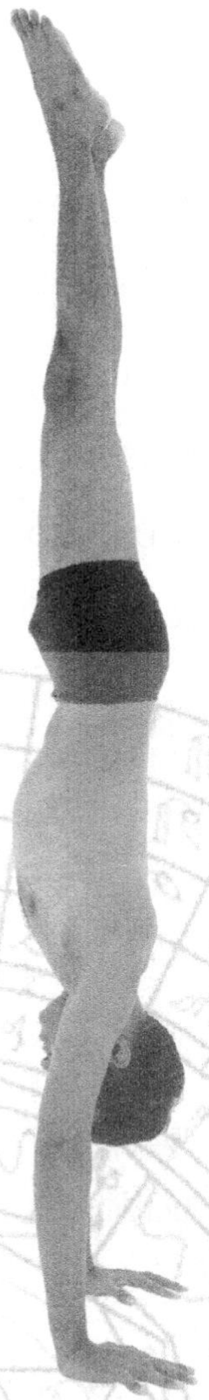

Figure: 282

Pranayamas:

Sitali Kapalabhati:

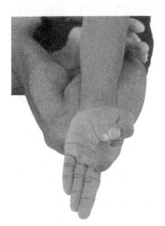
Figure: 283

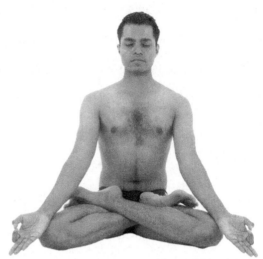
Figure: 284

How to enter:

Sit in sukasana or padmasana (Figure: 284). Keep your spine vertical and close your eyes. Place your hands in jnana mudra by bringing the tip of your index finger in contact with the tip of your thumb. Keep the remaining three fingers extended, yet relaxed (Figure: 283). Now place your palms up on your knees. Ensure you are comfortable so you can sit in this pose until the end of the pranayama practice. You may need to sit up on a block or bolster.

Bring the tip of your tongue on your lower lip, with your tongue a little bit out of your mouth, and keep your lips slightly open. Take a long inhale through the mouth, sending the air on the surface of your tongue, cooling your tongue. Then close your mouth and do a fast exhale through your nose while pulling your navel towards your spine. The diaphragm is pushed upwards. The velocity of the belly moving in is quite fast so the abdomen will bounce back to a neutral position by itself. Again, inhale slowly through the mouth and exhale strongly. Repeat this for 30 to 60 seconds effortlessly.

Once the practice is done, keep your breath passive and avoid over breathing.

Feel the passivity of your breath and experience the sensations inside your body. Feel the nerves relaxed and calm. As the breath becomes more passive, the brain receives a good oxygen supply, which helps to relieve stress and tension. This pranayama is remarkably helpful to cool your system from the heat that you created while doing the asana practice. Therefore, watch the sense of relaxation and dive deep into it.

Sitali Ujjayi Brahmari Ujjayi:

This is an advance pranayama. If you are a beginner with no background in doing any pranayama methods, then consult an experienced Universal Yoga® pranayama teacher. Only practice if you do not have any health condition that would be contraindicated to this technique. The reason it is kept in the advance category is mainly because you use bandhas (See Chapter 9 on bandhas). If you do not have experience practicing retentions of breath, then start your breathing practices slowly at first.

Once you have established your breathing patterns, then you can start retaining your breath for three to five seconds. If your pranayama practice gets deeper, then you can play with retentions of one or two minutes. As you progress even further, it is possible to hold even five minutes. In those moments activity becomes minimal and the thinking patterns will cease totally. It becomes natural and effortless. Once your practice advances enough, then you can do ujjayi pranayama and apply bandhas. This can uplift your energetic flow, and make your mind more clear and focused.

Here the term ujjayi has two stages, one is to retain the breath after inhalation, and the second stage is to retain the breath after exhalation.

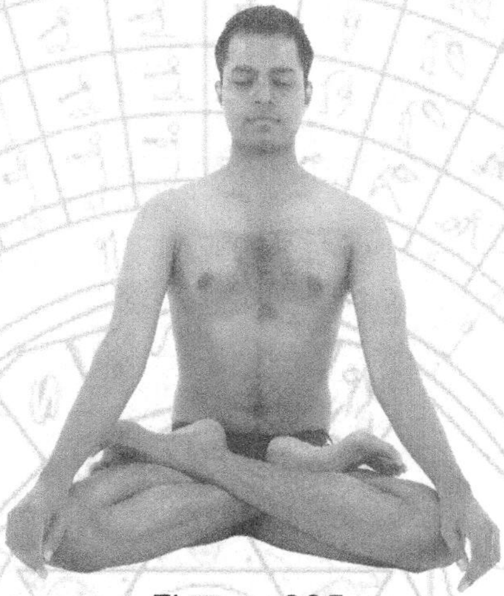

Figure: 285

How to enter:

Step 1:

Bring the tip of your tongue on your lower lip, with your tongue a little bit out of your mouth, and keep your lips slightly open. Take a long inhale through the mouth, sending the air on the surface of your tongue, cooling your tongue. Then close your mouth.

Step 2:

Gently hold your breath and perform mula bandha (pelvic floor) and jalandhara bandha (throat contraction) for five seconds.

Step 3:

Now close your mouth, relax your jaw, place your tongue on the back edge of your teeth, keep your lips gently closed, contract your glottis (the space between the vocal chords in your throat). Exhale slowly to create the sound of a bumble bee with an unobstructed rhythm. Keep the sound long and smooth. Feel the vibration around your abdomen, heart center, and in your head.

Step 4:

Now hold your breath again, and engage mula bandha (pelvic floor), uddiyana bandha (abdominal contraction), and jalandhara bandha (throat contraction) altogether. Hold for five seconds. This completes one round.

Slowly inhale repeating the steps six to ten more times. Once you have finished your pranayama session, uncross your legs, lay down on your back to prepare for shavasana.

Finishing pose:

Shavasana:

Shava: corpse. This pose is called corpse pose.

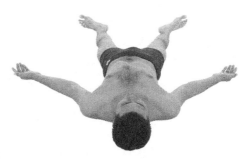

Figure: 286

Corpse pose is one of the unique poses in an asana practice. It's one of the essential methods to totally relax; particularly at the end of your asana session. During asana practice your sympathetic nervous system is activated. In order to compensate and balance your practice, you need to switch on your parasympathetic nervous system as well.

Rest in shavasana for at least 20-30 minutes to feel completely rejuvenated on the muscular, nervous system, and mental levels.

In yoga, stillness is one of the essential core practices that one has to encounter. After all of the sequential asana movements, it is easier to experience a state of stillness for a long period of time. This is why yoga practice is different from other fitness exercises. In yoga, after your physical practice you are allowing your body to be in a restful state. Your body can rest completely, yet you are awake inside. Shavasana helps you cease your brain activities. It helps to puts you in an alpha state. It's a very good beginning state, but our goal is to be more conscious and still, to get to what scientists call a delta state. That is where the frequency of your brain waves reduce to 0-4 cycles per second. Your body relaxes, but you are completely awake, without any ripples in your mind. Therefore, please do not skip shavansa practice after your asana practice. Practice until it becomes a very natural state within you.

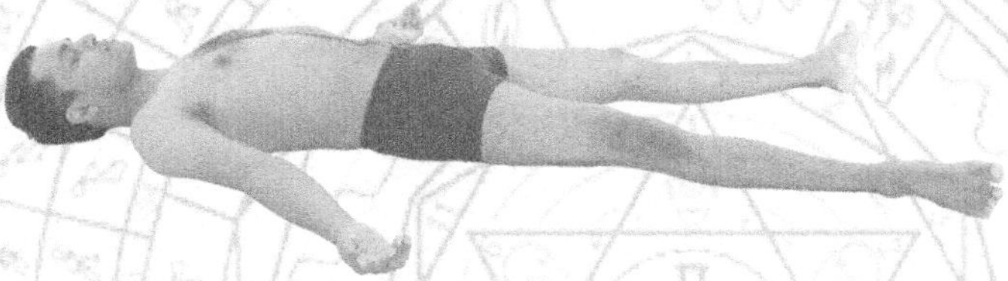

How to enter:

Lay on your back with your feet separated, keep your arms

Figure: 287

away from your torso, and keep your palms facing up with your fingers relaxed. Be still like a dead body (Figure: 286). Breathe freely, letting the breath become more passive as you relax. Notice if any tension is present in the body. Keep your forehead relaxed, eyes closed and relaxed. Keep your jaw relaxed, your tongue rests on the bottom of the mouth. See if any tension is present on the surface. If the body starts fidgeting, relax more and don't fidget. Keep your breath passive and nonagitated; let it move naturally and avoid over breathing (Figure: 287).

Your breath can fall back into its own nature, therefore don't alter your breathing pattern. When you become aware of your breath, the breath ratio might increase. Stop this ratio and be more passive in your breathing.

Now become aware of your whole body and find stillness from within. Notice if any thoughts are floating, avoid controlling the thoughts. If the thoughts are floating, notice that they are there, let them be there, and eventually you can create a gap between you and your thoughts. In that moment you will experience a glimpse of stillness.

Again we may fall into the clutches of moods and emotions, be aware of them. Through gradual practice you can overcome emotional patterns. Sometimes good thoughts will come and sometimes bad thoughts will appear, just watch, and stop all judgmental conversations. Become nonjudgmental and rest for at least 20-30 minutes.

To release, move your fingers and toes. Bring your arms over your head and stretch deeply. Bend your knees and rock up to a seated position.

Meditation:

Kaivalya:

How to enter:

Find a comfortable seated position that you can stay in for a fair amount of time like sukhasana or padmasana (Figure: 288).

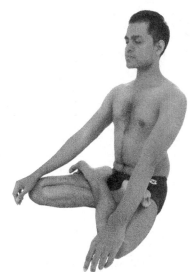

Figure: 288

In order to experience a vast infinite state of stillness, your body must be prepared to be still after all of the movements the body experienced in the asana practice. Here the mind is neither in the past nor in the future, but totally fixed in the present moment where the mind is not a barrier anymore. In those moments, you can feel the distance between you and your body. You can feel the distance between you and your mind very clearly.

Eventually, your attention to the present moment will be established well. Those moments are what you will look forward to in the process of a yogic practice. It is not the asanas that make a yoga practitioner look great. It is not the pranayama that makes a practitioner feel good. But an inbetween stage, a union between both. That understanding will not make a person want to escape from life, rather it helps them live life to the fullest; to the optimum level possible. Eventually one will realize that all methods, techniques, and technology of yoga is built up for the sake of humanity to rediscover this forgotten path.

You might use asana, pranayama, mantra, prayer, or religion. If you find that inner path, you will not exclude any technique. You will play with all sorts of techniques and enjoy the flow of the current. This is what we call kaivalya. A state of emancipation.

Mantras:

Sit in sukasana or padmasana with hands in namaste mudra (Figure: 289).

Karmic Purification Mantra:

Om Namo Bhagavate

Salutation to god

Sumeru Kalparajya

King who is the beginning and end of time on Mt. Meru

Tatyagataya

Liberated one

Arhate samek sambuddhaya

Spiritual warrior who conquers all negative karma

Taddyatham

So I'm talking

Om kalpe kalpe maha kalpe

I pray for the times, times and great times,

Praishodhani- svahamm-m

Of complete purification.

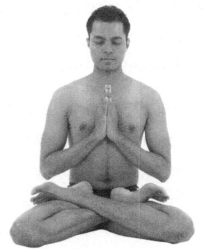

Figure: 289

Dedication Mantra:

I dedicate the merit of my practice,

To the spiritual liberation of all living beings,

By this merit may I quickly reach enlightenment,

And may I lead all living beings,

Without any exclusions,

To the same state of consciousness.

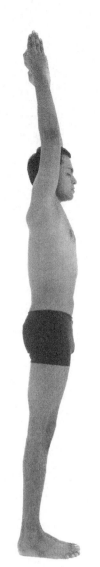

Ending:

Short Prostration:

Stand in tadasana, keep your feet together, arms resting next to thighs. As you inhale, raise your arms up over your head, and place your palms together (Figure: 290).

As you exhale, fold forward, bend your knees, and place you knees, palms, and forehead on the floor (Figure: 291).

Stretch your arms out and prostrate to the universe, and to your teacher (Figure: 292). This is a gesture of complete surrender to the universe and to the creator.

Bend your elbows (Figure: 291), as you inhale raise your head and stand up with your arms over your head again (Figure: 290). When you exhale bring your palms together at your heart center.

Figure: 290

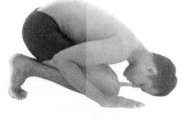

Figure: 291

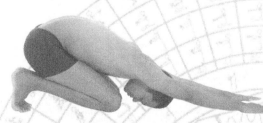

Figure: 292

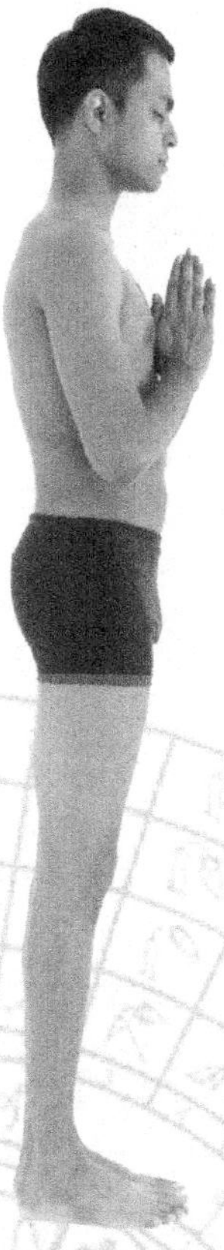

Figure: 293

This concludes the 4x4 Universal Yoga® Mandala Sequence.

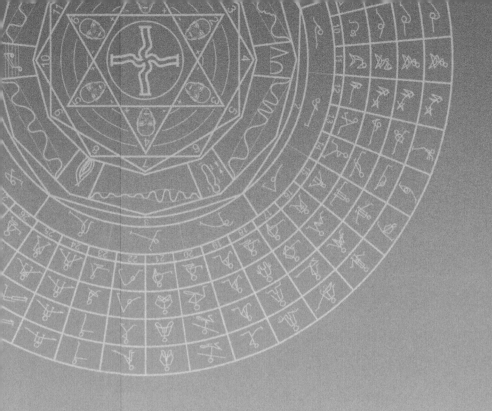

CHAPTER 9

Pranayama, Mudras, and Bandhas

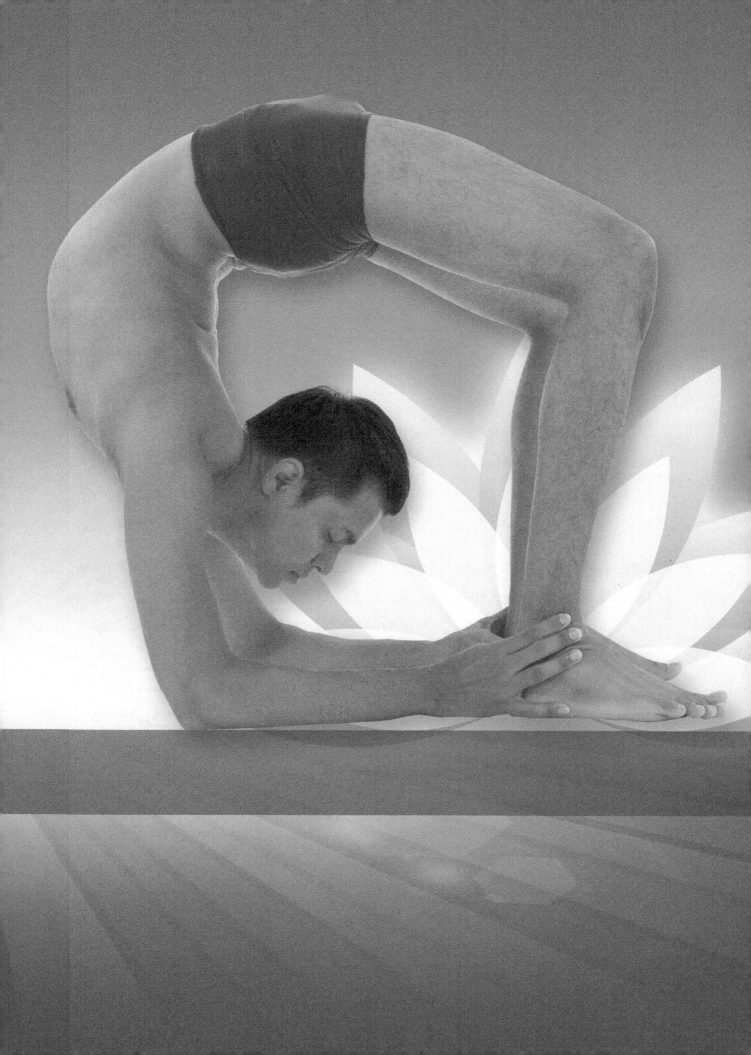

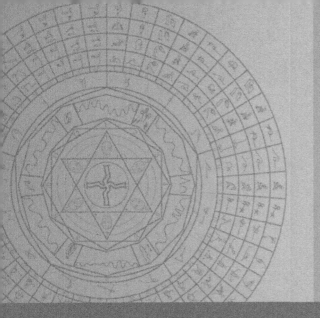

CHAPTER 9

Pranayama, Mudras, and Bandhas

Pranayama is an important tool that can be a direct bridge to the mind. The level of inhalation and exhalation should be slow and steady until it reaches its full capacity. Oxygen, which is a fundamental gas needed for the whole organism to continue to live, comes into the body through the lungs.

When we breathe through the nose, the nostril passages are filled with a mucus membrane that keeps the passage moist. This filters heavy particles, preventing them from entering the lungs. When the air passes through the lungs, the oxygen moves into the bloodstream and travels throughout the body. Here the oxygen cells are exchanged for waste gases called carbon dioxide. The bloodstream then carries the unwanted gas back to the lungs, where the waste gas is removed from the bloodstream. It is then released through the exhale. These actions happen in the respiratory system involuntarily. Therefore, it is important to breathe through the nose, not through the mouth. Certain breathing techniques are done through the mouth, but discuss this with your Universal Yoga® teacher for further clarification.

Here, pranayama plays a major role in overcoming certain respiratory disorders. Poor posture can cause breathing trouble. With regular practice and a moderate diet using strict discipline, one may overcome respiratory issues. During inhalation, the intercostal muscles contract helping to activate the ribcage. The diaphragm moves down and that causes the lower ribs to expand, allowing the abdominal organs to move downward and forward. During exhalation, the intercostal muscles relax. As the ribcage moves back and down, and as the diaphragm relaxes, the volume of the chest decreases. However, the pressure in the chest increases and thus helps the air move out of the lungs eventually. Yoga mainly emphasizes a consciously controlled breath.

Today's lifestyle is fast paced and everything is swift, so many people do not breathe deeply. If the lifestyle is going fast and quick, breath becomes shallow. In a busy lifestyle, one finishes work, goes home, becomes very lethargic, has dinner, and moves to a drowsy state. This poor lifestyle will unconsciously accumulate more poison in the body! That is why yoga is a treasure, particularly for the one who lives this type of sedentary lifestyle. Pranayama proposes a consciously controlled breath that ultimately leads to a healthy lifestyle.

Movement of the Breath During Asana:

When practicing the 4 x 4 Universal Yoga® Mandala sequence, one should maintain so-ham pranayama. So-ham is one of the old, traditional ways of practice, and as such it can also be used as a mantra. You can repeat "so-ham" while you hold each asana, maintaining an equal ratio of inhale ("so") and exhale ("ham"). When it is done in this way, it is no longer just physical practice but an internal practice that helps one achieve a concentrated state of mind. This state of mind helps your dhyana (meditation) practice to be more active. It is an important technique of breathing that many schools have emphasized.

When you practice asanas with vinyasa, your breath should be more calm and steady. Hold your postures for six breaths minimum in each pose. If your practice is established then you can hold each pose for 12 to 16 breaths. The breath should neither be erratic nor shallow while you are holding the pose. It is common to breathe erratically when you do some complex asanas. It might even be harder to breathe at all in the beginning. First apply a slow and steady breath in the simple asanas. As your body reacts to your practice, then apply more complex movements, but try to maintain a deep relaxation in your body and breath. Avoid making an exaggerated breath, which makes a heavy sound and noise. This can sometimes cause tiredness or even a light-headed sensation. Applying gentle pressure to your practice can make your practice more steady and joyful. Experience this sequence and reach an optimum level of benefits from this great practice.

Pranayamas after Asana:

In Universal Yoga®, we have a wide range of breathing techniques that are quite creative and rebellious. They bring a new revolution to those who have practiced the same pranayamas for many years. It is not that the old has to be changed to bring the new in. The Universal Yoga® prototype breathing techniques are absolutely taken from the traditional hatha yoga practices themselves. Therefore, there is nothing to be afraid of regarding these breathing techniques. After years of practice, Andrey Lappa has discovered that these techniques not only give a strong effect to the nervous system, but they also help to deeply pacify the mind.

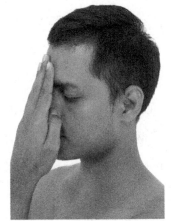

1. Sitali Chandra Bhedana Pranayama
How to enter:
Sit in padmasana (lotus posture). Place the four fingers of your right hand on your forehead and your right thumb

Figure: 9.1

on your right nostril to close it (Figure 9.1). Keep your left hand in jnana mudra on your left knee with your palm facing up (Figure 9.2). Bring the tip of your tongue on your lower lip, with your tongue a little bit out of your mouth, and keep your lips slightly open. Breathe in through the mouth, sending the air on the surface of your tongue, cooling your tongue. Then close your mouth and exhale through your left open nostril. This is one round. Once you maintain this breath pattern uninterrupted with proper coordination, then repeat for six rounds.

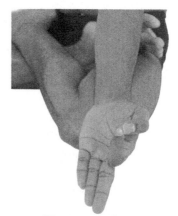

Figure: 9.2

2. Sitali Surya Bhedana Pranayama

How to enter:

Sit in padmasana (lotus posture). Place the four fingers of your left hand on your forehead and the left thumb on your left nostril to close it (Figure 9.1). Keep your right hand in jnana mudra on your right knee with your palm facing up (Figure 9.2). Bring the tip of your tongue on your lower lip, with your tongue a little bit out of your mouth, and keep your lips slightly open. Breathe in through the mouth, sending the air on the surface of your tongue, cooling your tongue. Then close your mouth and exhale through your right open nostril. This is one round. Once you can maintain this breath pattern uninterrupted with proper coordination, then repeat for six rounds.

3. Sitali Kapalbhati:

How to enter:

Sit in sukhasana or padmasana. Keep your back upright and close your eyes gently. Place your hands in jnana mudra (Figure:

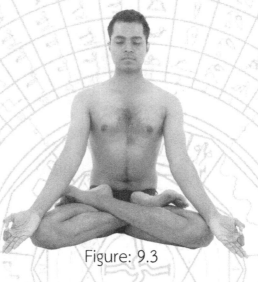

Figure: 9.3

9.3). Connect your thumb and index finger together and keep your other fingers straight and relaxed with palms facing up on your knees. Ensure you can sit in this pose until the end of the pranayama practice. Be comfortable.

Bring the tip of your tongue on your lower lip, with your tongue a little bit out of your mouth, and keep your lips slightly open. Breathe in through the mouth, sending the air on the surface of your tongue, cooling your tongue. Then close your mouth, exhale fast, and pull your navel towards your spine. The diaphragm is pushed upwards. Here the velocity of the belly moving in is quite fast. Let the abdomen bounce back to a neutral position by itself while inhaling slowly through the mouth again. Then repeat the strong exhale through the nostrils. Continue this technique for 30 to 60 seconds effortlessly.

4. Sitali Ujjayi Sitali Bhramari Ujjayi:

How to enter:

Step 1:

Sit in padmasana (Figure: 9.5). Hands are in jnana mudra, palms facing up (Figure: 9.4). Unclench your jaw and teeth. Bring the tip of your tongue on your lower lip, with your tongue a little bit out of your mouth, and keep your lips slightly open. Breathe in through the mouth, sending the air on the surface of your tongue, cooling your tongue. Inhale a long, slow breath through your mouth. Keep your

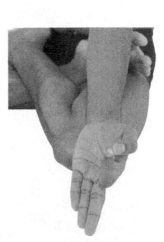

Figure: 9.4

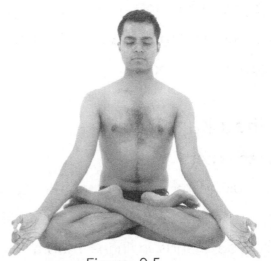

Figure: 9.5

lungs, chest, and ribs active. Once you inhale fully, hold your breath and maintain the breath retention with mula bandha and jalandhara bandha (see bandha topic in this chapter). Hold each retention for 5 to 8 seconds.

Note:

In Universal Yoga®, we call these bandhas with retentions as ujjayi, hence the name of the pranayama. It is one of the ancient traditional practices. Where ujjayi has been maintained in this order, ujjayi is not just a victorious breath, but a combination of so-ham pranayama along with bandhas together.)

Step 2:

As you exhale, close your mouth and relax your jaw. Place the tip of the tongue on the front edge of the teeth. Keep your lips gently closed. Contract your glottis (the space between the vocal cords in your throat). As you breathe out through the nose, create the sound of a bumble bee with an unobstructed rhythm. Keep the sound long and smooth. You will feel the vibration around your abdomen, heart center, and in your head as well. Maintain the brahmari (bumble bee) sound until the air is released from the lungs.

Step 3:

Hold your breath again by contracting mula bandha (the pelvic floor), uddiyana bandha (the abdominal contraction), and jalandhara bandha (the throat contraction) simultaneously. Hold for five seconds. This is one round. Inhale and repeat the same for 6 to 10 rounds.

Mudras:

In Sanskrit, mudra means "a seal of energy".

Mudras are specific gestures that are mainly used in asana, pranayama, and meditation. In this sequence you will have specific mudras during asana and pranayama that can help create an energetic influence on the body. Joining the fingers with different coordinated positions create balance in the human body.

Mudras are done with the hands, legs, and through postures also. Mudras were used as a traditional part of Indian dance (Bharatanatyam) to express the feelings and thoughts of the dancers. The gestures were also a part of the traditional Indian and Buddhist practices. Mudras can also be used for healing purposes. In the 4 x 4 Universal Yoga® Mandala sequence, we have four main hand gestures.

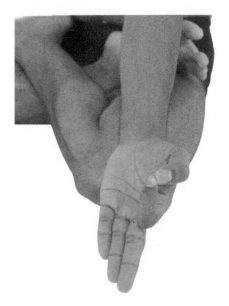

Jnana Mudra:

In Sanskrit, jnana means "knowledge". It is knowledge through self-realization.

Relax your hands and bring the tip of your index finger in contact with the tip of your thumb. Keep the remaining three fingers extended, yet relaxed (Figure: 9.6).

Figure: 9.6

Namaste/Namaskar Mudra (also called Anjali Mudra):

Bend your elbows. Bring both hands and palms together at the center of the chest with the fingers facing upward. Keep your thumbs close to the heart center (Figure: 9.7). The word namaste or namaskar means "I bow to you" in the context that everyone is equal and there is nothing such as "mine". This idea of having for myself can be demolished from the mind. Thinking of myself is bondage and having an attitude of nothing as mine is freedom. Hence, this gesture is very important. If this gesture is done mechanically, then there is no purpose to using this gesture at all. For centuries in India, people have used this method for a simple reason. In yoga, we see this gesture in its broader aspect.

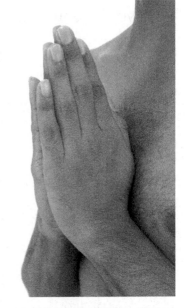

Figure: 9.7

Mushti Mudra:

In Sanskrit, mushti means "fist".

Relax your hands and place your thumb inside the edge of your ring finger and close your four fingers over the thumb. Slightly clench your fingers and form a shape of mushti (Figure: 9.8). This mudra helps provoke heat in the wrist and

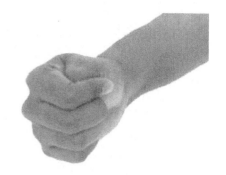

Figure: 9.8

activates blood flow around the arms and hands. This can also be done to release negative emotions, when the body has a tendency to react to emotional changes. Since part of the energy is accumulated in the hands, teeth, and legs, a part of the gesture can be practiced separately by clenching the fist in order to eliminate particular emotional blockages.

Vishnu Mudra:

This mudra can be practiced during any pranayama method in the Universal Yoga® system where you are inhaling through one nostril and exhaling through the other. Relax your hands. Bend your ring and little fingers placing your thumb over them. Extend the index and middle fingers together (Figure: 9.9). This is a meditative method that helps fix the mind at one point, steadily.

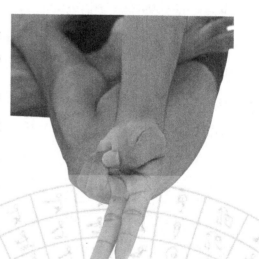

Figure: 9.9

Bandhas:

Bandhas are one of the important chapters in the hatha yoga tradition. Bandhas are not mentioned in *Yoga Sutras of Patanjali*, but in the hatha yoga lineage, they are essential techniques to activate the sushumna channel. These methods are not advisable for beginning practitioners nor for those needing therapeutic techniques. If one has established a good range of mobility in their asana practice and a good range of breath in their pranayama practice, then it is preferable to introduce bandhas into the regular practice. This is particularly true for one who is able to maintain soft, long breaths without any difficulty, and for one who can retain the breath while maintaining a tranquil nervous system.

Bandhas help to unlock your nadis (channels). They also help improve blood flow in those channels as long as the body is prepared enough to handle these pressures. When you begin, it is perfectly fine to apply locks and retentions for shorter periods of time. As you evolve, you can play with these techniques for longer periods of time and in deeper ways. When I say "play with these techniques", I don't mean that you should practice like you are playing games. Rather, I want you to practice these methods regularly and in a serious way. The kind of interest will help you to attain the state of the result. Again, yoga practice is not a result-oriented method. Therefore, practice without expecting any results. This is the way to not have frustrations. Rather, you surrender to the moment when you involve yourself into these practices.

The very word bandha means "to lock", "to tighten", "to arrest" and "to restrain". You apply a certain pressure on a particular area of the body by using breath retention. This helps produce a powerful energetic effect increasing the flow of energy into the main channel called sushumna nadi. It can have an effect on the physical body, energetic body, and psychic body as well.

In the West, it is currently very popular to say "use the pelvic floor" during asana practice. This is not the same as using bandhas. As we know that true bandhas are used specifically in static positions while retaining the breath. More specifically, they are practiced to awaken the energy called kundalini.

During asana practice, if you always apply the pelvic floor lock, it is not going to make your postures relaxed and steady, as Patanjali has mentioned in his yoga sutra (stira sukham asanam). Rather, this causes one to apply more pressure in the pose, leading to a tendency to over tense the muscles and over breathe in the pose. That is not a good way to practice. The East proposes that we practice yoga in another way. If you practice the Western way, you might be able to do the posture and you will look good in the asana, but the main purpose of the bandha is missed. If one tends to contract the root and navel most of the time, especially during the time when one is no longer doing any postures, then we can say that such a practice is not right.

Let's make it clear that using bandhas might be good if one is sick or unable to do things. In day-to-day life, it is perfectly fine to use these bandhas for therapeutic purposes and under any critical conditions. But the bandhas do not affect only the physical or psychic parts of the body. In order to gain the maximum result, you need to apply bandhas before meditation. If bandhas are reduced to usefulness only during asana, then the purpose and the real value of doing the bandhas will be left behind. It is not necessary to do bandhas all the time. Once your body adapts to these practices, you will enjoy using them during the particular time when they are needed. You will also know when to drop the techniques. Real liberation happens only when you drop all the techniques which were given to you to attain the ultimate path.

There are many types of bandhas we can perform in our body. According to *Hatha Yoga Pradipika*, there are three important bandhas to be performed. It is said in ancient texts, that these bandhas can help to overcome one's old age and even death.

At first, it is helpful to learn them one after the other. Once you have learned the way to hold these bandhas separately, then you can practice them together, as we have explained in this Universal Yoga® system of practice.

- Jalandhara Bandha: Throat Lock
- Uddiyana Bandha: Navel Lock
- Mula Bandha: Anus and Pelvic Floor Lock
- Maha Bandha: Combination of all Three locks together

1. Jalandhara Bandha:

Jalandhara means "upward pulling net" or "net in the stream".

In order to engage this bandha, sit in any meditative pose. As you inhale, round your neck and press the chin firmly against the chest or between the collarbones so that the windpipe and esophagus are firmly closed. Hold for five seconds with a relaxed state of mind, and when you exhale, release the lock gently. Relax your neck and shoulders. This is one round. If you establish this method fairly well, then increase the duration of the hold. Also perform this lock after your exhale and hold. This is the next stage of the bandha that you should practice doing until you are able to perform it without any difficulties.

2. Uddiyana Bandha:

The word uddiyana means "to raise".

In the beginning, it is good to practice this bandha in a standing pose as a sitting position is often harder. As you progress, if you know how to do it in a standing position, then use a sitting position. Through regular practice, you will be able to easily perform the bandha in a seated position.

Before practicing uddiyana bandha, be sure that you are able to perform jalandhara bandha very well. In uddiyana, you must invariably access your jalandhara bandha as well. During uddiyana practice, if a student is too relaxed on the throat center, which is the jalandhara bandha part, then the pressure which is cultivated from the bottom can be pushed upward without any control. This results in high volume pressure and leads to lightheadedness, black out, or even death.

Now let's see how to perform uddiyana bandha in a sitting position. Sit in a comfortable meditation position. Inhale completely. As you exhale, empty the lungs and hold the breath. Pull the abdominal muscles toward the spine and expand the ribcage, thus helping to raise the diaphragm up. Here, you act as if you are inhaling, but you don't actually inhale. Instead, press your chin to the chest and expand the chest up while you hold the belly in. This will stop the air from entering. Ensure that the abdomen muscles are not contracted too tight. Do not apply any tension on the muscles. Rather, keep the belly muscles soft and relaxed. Hold for five to ten seconds. Right before you inhale, release the neck and relax the abdomen. This is one round. As you progress, you can practice twenty-five rounds without straining the body. Avoid practicing this method during menstruation or pregnancy. The best time to practice is early in the morning on an empty stomach.

3. Mula Bandha:

Mula means "root". It is often called "pelvic floor" or "root lock".

Sit in a comfortable position, keeping the body upright and erect. Place the palms on the knees. Avoid tension in your body. As you inhale, bring your chin to the chest in jalandhara bandha and contract the perineum. Draw the pelvic floor up toward the navel; this includes contracting ashvini (anus), yoni (perineal/

cervix), and vajroli (urethra) mudras at the same time. Do not contract the gluteus muscles. For a male, yoni mudra is situated between the anus and the genitals, the perineal region. For a female, it is situated at the cervix. Avoid forceful contractions, as this is not advisable. Stay and engage the bandha for 5 to 10 seconds, then exhale. This is one round. You can repeat this method as many times as you want.

Maha Bandha:

Maha means "great". When you combine these three bandhas together it becomes maha bandha (the great lock). In the 4 x 4 Universal Yoga® Mandala sequence, you will perform these three locks (mula, uddiyana, and jalandara bandhas) together towards the end of the practice. You inhale, hold the breath, and lock these three bandhas together. Then you exhale, release the bandhas, then hold the breath out and engage the three bandhas together. This will be one round.

Maha Bandha

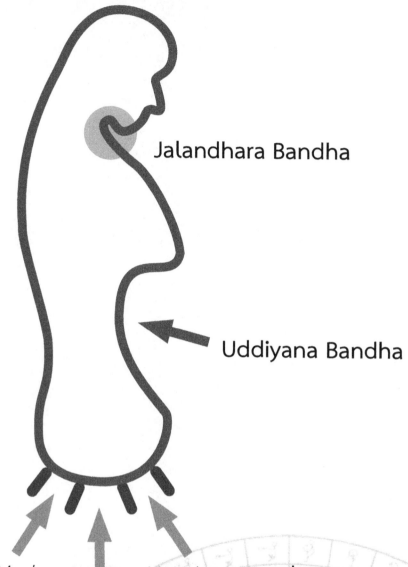

Jalandhara Bandha

Uddiyana Bandha

Ashvini Mudra

Yoni Mudra

Vajroli Mudra

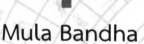

Mula Bandha

Figure: 9.10

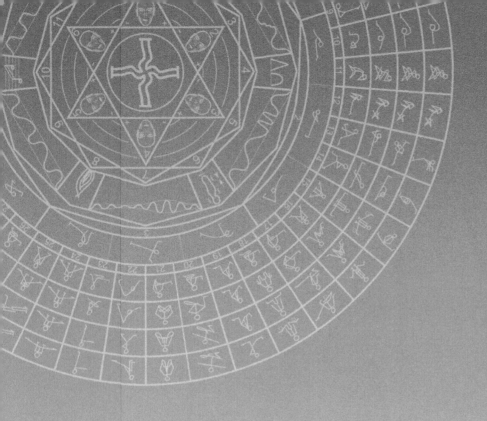

CHAPTER 10

Road to Kaivalya

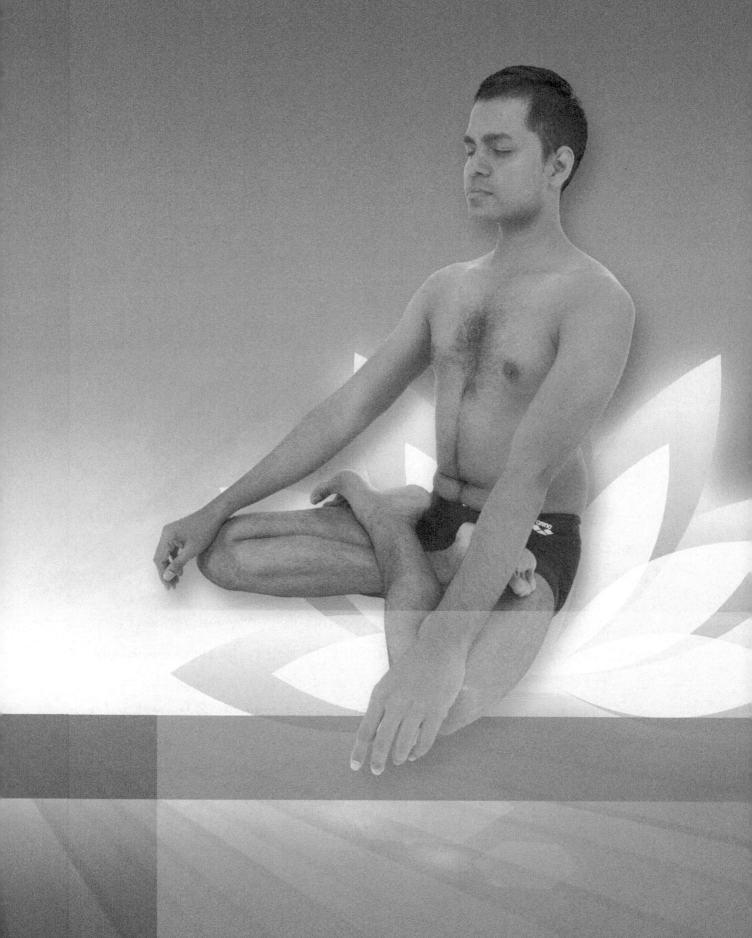

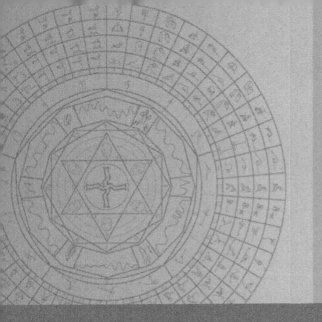

CHAPTER 10

Road to Kaivalya

The mind is a complex and wonderful gadget, yet constantly being in connection with the mind is an imprisonment. Knowing the mind and acting through your own awareness is the goal of yoga.

Mind is constantly anchored in an unconscious state. It anchors us down in the form of desires, ego, anger, jealousy, name, fame, prestige, power trips, social status, passion, and ambitions. Consequently, one may perceive life as misery.

Yoga was not designed as a means to make this life happy. Remember, Patanjali never mentioned the bringing of happiness in. Rather, he proposed a way for us to get out of the samsara (vicious cycle of life and death) of life! He is not proposing that we live forever either. Rather, he explains how to deal with our sufferings! As you overcome the suffering, the joy of life happens, which is eternal. It is like dark clouds are obstructing the sunshine, and as the clouds disperse, the rays of light come to the flowers, your balcony, your room, or the place where you sleep. It simply follows you instantaneously.

Yoga is about how to promote your body and mind to the optimum level. As it is said in the *Yoga Vasistha*, an ancient Sanskrit text: "For the ignorant person, this body is the source of endless suffering, but to the wise person, this body is the source of infinite delight."

Yoga is not about doing postures and some breath retention exercises. Yoga is a complete alchemical knowledge that can turn bronze into gold. It is turning totally inward. It is neither moving to the past nor the future, but surrendering completely to this moment!

If you overcome your rapidly flowing thoughts, you are in yoga. Some people get to the state of silence by praying to Jesus Christ, Muhammad or another figure or entity. It is not a question of which technique you follow. There are many techniques! Similarly, there can be many religions, but the goal is the same. At its simplest, yoga gives us a unified form. Compiled together it says if you follow the way with trust, you can attain the goal. There were many who set themselves free from the negative patterns of the mind. Now let's look into the four states of mind.

Four States of Mind:

Waking State (Jagrat):

Day-to-day life is experienced through this state. One is in a permanent connection with the sensory organs—the jnanendriyas (ears, eyes, nose, tongue, and skin). This is where the mind function becomes predominant and one identifies with the ego, intelligence and memory.

Dreaming State (Swapna):

The second state is a little deeper, where one stores unwanted thoughts and suppressed emotions that can pop up when in a dream state; when the subconscious memory starts functioning more.

Deep Sleeping State (Sushupti):

The third layer is deep sleep state or unconscious state where one enters deep sleep. In this state there is no function of ego or dreams. One forgets oneself and the conscious state does not exist. It's like being transported into another world, yet unaware of what is happening, as if in a trance, yet unconscious of what being in a trance means.

Super Conscious State (Turiya):

A pure awareness state, or supraconscious state. One is in a state of advaita (non-duality), neither judging nor discriminating but in a state of awakening. The mind is no more a master, but one knows how to use the mind more effectively. This is a state where mind functioning has ceased. In this state transformation happens.

Most of the time one lives in the waking state (jagrat) or in a dream state (swapna). The state of one's mind is the gateway for suffering. Man has learned to be in suffering through unconscious activities, as if giving more importance to the mind, but not to the observer (the true Self).

Is our mind the master or is one's true Self the master? This reminds me of a story I've loved since first hearing it. Let me share the story of Mohamed Farid.

The Mohamed Farid Story

One afternoon, Farid was passing through a village. He saw a man who had tied a rope to his cow and was taking the cow to his house. Farid said to his disciples, "Go and surround this man and his cow. I want to teach you something!"

The man was a little startled. He said, "Why are you surrounding me?"

Farid said, "We aren't concerned with you, but I want to teach to my disciples."

So, he asked his disciples, "Of these two, a man and a cow, who is the master?"

The disciples said, "What are you asking? It's quite clear that the man is the master because the cow is his property, and he has a tied rope around the cow's neck."

Farid said, "I will ask you a second question. Suppose we cut the rope and the cow runs away, will the cow follow the man or will the man follow the cow?"

The disciples replied, "Certainly it is the man who will run after the cow."

"So, this means the cow will not go searching for the man? The man will search for the cow? If this is the situation, then who is the master?"

Mastering Oneself:

Most people always want to achieve something, constantly running after the achievement. The beauty of a yogic attitude is not to master things but to master oneself.

If you are in the field of yoga, it is not that you are achieving the postures; rather, you are disciplining your body and passing through the state of the body's old habits. As you evolve more, you are no more in the circumference of the body. Instead, you go deeper into the realm of the infinite source. In order to move away from this circumference, one has to find out his range of interest.

Your range of interest can begin with religion. Religion was built to create a discipline for oneself. Instead, we try to push it onto others to follow the same morality that perhaps you were forced to follow. Every religion has contributed something to this planet. If one is wakeful enough, one can see the reasons underlying these religious functions that can influence each of us.

The yogic revolution did not begun through religion, although religion can be a starting point for yoga to be discovered. The aim of these revolutionary acts is to awaken one's inner potential. When you are in search of the internal, the path is seen. You are no longer interested in the outer. It is at that moment that yoga works as a quantum leap. With a sudden change in your gesture, you can see old habits and attitudes wither away, and something new born out of it.

With that burning desire, one functions from a deep awareness with a full possibility for attainment.

When you become more profound and tangible, only then are you living in the dimension of yoga. A new quality is born out of it. In order to attain this new beginning, one should have an interest. It is not an interest in the outer, but of the internal. The interest can vary from person to person. Buddha simplified it clearly as finding out your range of interests. The size of your leap into yoga will vary according to your interests.

Let's see the interest levels that can be used as a map to understand the quality of your yogic journey.

Three types of interest to attain the quality of your inner growth;

Kutuhal (Interest, Eager)

Some people enter into yoga class just to get superficial results, because many people assume that being fit and firm means they are very healthy. At that stage, one doesn't understand the secret of a healthy mind.

First, in order to drop the mind, the mind should be healthy. Only a healthy mind can understand the idea of dropping the mind. Remember here, the mind initiates the drop of the mind. Therefore, the mind should be healthy.

For the kutuhal seeker, however, it is not the main concern. Their concern is mainly to be slim and strong. Their lifestyle will not change much. Here, they might get the idea of enlightenment or moksha, but not much work is done to initiate the process, because the purification process is not deep. The vrttis (fluctuations) of the mind and the vasanas (sensory pleasures) drag them to the same old habits of samskaras; they go nowhere. Rather, they are stuck in the same place where they started. It is simply a matter of being curious about changing the body but not ready to invest all of one's energy into the goal of ultimate growth.

Jigyasa (Analysis, Research)

The jigyasa seekers invest some energy into ultimate growth. The process of searching begins here, and they understand that just by practicing asana and pranayama, one cannot attain the higher goal. Therefore, they start to examine yoga more closely. It is something like being half asleep but also half awake. Something triggers a desire to learn more. It might be because of losing a loved one or because all your desires have been fulfilled. Yet a feeling of emptiness lingers inside. Or they simply trust their guru to help them become awakened. Therefore, the thirst for knowledge gets deeper. Such students start to examine the ancient Vedic knowledge more extensively. But this is not enough. It is still just a search. It is not a complete transformation, and many are stuck here because they research so much but never put their knowledge into actual practice. You can see people saying that they know what you ask them to do, but they never actually practice and gain experience. If the seed of knowledge is impotent, then the tree of wisdom does not grow.

Mumuksha (Burning Desire to Attain Enlightenment)

Ego is fallible. Ego wants to hold the outer power. As long as one is under the clutches of the mind, tethered here and there, the mind doesn't know where to start and where to end. This in turn brings misery to life. If the ego prevents you from doing something new, use the new-found knowledge to defeat your own ego. Hence, the ego brings all sorts of shortcuts to divert you from reaching the inner world. Buddha taught that if you just have curiosity, it is not going to fulfill your life. Rather, a burning desire is needed. Only an urge is needed to reach the ultimate. The very readiness of transformation can help you attain the goal.

The will of the mumuksha seeker has to be strong and unobstructed. Then the burning desire will guide one to the new height. It is not the regular desire which usually leads one's life into misery. It is a disturbed passion that won't let you sleep properly or work properly. Each time you find rest, the burning desire will shake you up. It is not the question of attaining the goal, because the urge to search is very strong. It will definitely lead you to the right path. But only sincere spiritual investigation, with strong passion, can give the seeker the desire to search for a real guru to help teach them the way. Only then is it possible to dissolve into nothingness.

Here Kabir explains!
Kabir says,
"Oh! my friend! Seeking and searching, Kabir has been dissolved."
(The Kabir Book, The Ecstatic Songs of Kabir)

The path is exactly the same here; be a mumuksha to be a strong seeker. Only then will transformation happen totally. Only then does the old self disappear and the true being starts to emerge. Here the seeking is absolutely necessary to reach the state of non-seeking. Be a mumuksha and it's a sure way to transform oneself successfully.

Sanskrit Glossary

A

Abhika	being affectionate, caring
Abhyasa	constant practice, dedication
Adi Yogi	first yogi (yogi who discovered the path of liberation)
Advaita	nonduality
Agni	fire
Ahamkara	the ego function
Ahimsa	non-violence
Ajna	sixth chakra situated in between the eyebrow
Anahtata	heart chakra situated behind the chest
Ananda	state of supreme bliss
Anapana	conscious breath flow of inhalation and exhalation
Anjali Mudra	prayer gesture (hands together and fingers facing upward)
Anuloma	in the natural rhythm or flow, with the hair
Apana	downward flow of breath
Aparigraha	non-greediness
Arhat	one who is ready or pregnant to attain the state of liberation
Asana	a steady and comfortable position of the body, third limb of ashtanga yoga
Ashtanga	limbed path designed by sage Patanjali
Asteya	non-stealing
Atharva Veda	fourth veda "alter"
Atman	pure self, soul

Avidhya	ignorance
Ayurveda	science of life, holistic way of life, another great discovery by Maharishi Patanjali

B

Baddha	bound
Baka	crane
Bala	child
Bandhas	lock of energy
Bhagavad Gita	5000 years old ancient story designed as "a song of god", the story of Arjuna, a warrior, who is taught by his charioteer, Krishna
Bhajan	a hymn
Bhakti Yoga	devotion, a school that emphasizes surrender to god
Bhavana	attitude
Bhodi	enlightened
Bhoga	enjoyment, indulge in sensory pleasure
Bhuta	elements
Bhuva	earth
Brahma muhurta	an auspicious time to wake up and meditate
Brahmacharya	chastity
Brahmari	bumble bee sound
Buddha	an awakened being
Buddhi	intelligence
Bhuja	arm

C

Chakra	wheel

D

Danda	staff
Dhyana	yantra
Dukha	suffering
Dwi	two

E

Eka Grata	one pointedness
Eka	one

G

Garuda	eagle
Guru	a teacher, one who illuminates light on his disciples

H

Hala	plough
Hanumana	name of monkey deity
Hasta	hand
Hatha	Hatha refers to "force" or "fierce" discipline, which born as a pashupatha yoga, a strong ascetic tantric practice to attain the ultimate liberation

I

Indriya	sensory organ
Isa	lord

J

Jagrat	waking state
Jalandhara	a method to lock your neck and throat

Janu	knee
Japa	repetitive prayer
Jigyasa	curiosity to know
Jivatma	soul of each individual person

K

Kaivalya	an ultimate emancipation
Kapota	pigeon
Karuna	compassion (unconditional love)
Kurma	tortoise
Kuthukal	superficial interest

M

Maitri	friendship
Mandala	matrix symbol
Manduka	frog
Manipura	situated behind the navel
Matsyendra	fish
Moksha	liberation
Muladhara	first chakra, situated at the base of the spine
Mudra	a seal of energy
Mula Bandha	a method to lock the perineum and lifted up towards the spine

N

Namaskar	Indian way of greetings with utmost respect

P

Pada	foot
Padma	lotus
Paripurna	complete

Parsva	side
Patanjali	a sage who was born approximately 500-200 BCE and author of *Yoga Sutras of Patanjali*
Pratiloma	opposite of the natural rhythm "opposite the hair"
Puja	worship or prayer
Purusha	uncontaminated conscious being

R

Raga	attachment, anger, passion
Rajas	hyperactivity, overactive

S

Sahasrara	crown chakra situated on the crown of the head
Salabha	locust
Samadhi	a state of enlightenment
Samskara	an embedded impression
Santosa	contentment, deep gratitude towards life
Sattva	luminosity, purity
Satya	truth
Saucha	cleanliness
Setu	bridge
Shavasana	corpse
Sheath	shells
Siddhi	occult power
Sirsa	head
Sitali	one of the cooling pranayama
Surya	sun
Svana	dog
Swadhistana	situated in the spine above genitals.
Swadhyaya	self-study by noticing one's own life

T

Tada	mountain
Tamas	dullness, darkness
Tantra	technique to awake the super consciousness
Tapas	strict ascetic discipline
Tri	three

U

Uddiyana Bandha	abdominal contraction, it is done by pulling the navel towards the spine
Ujjayi	one of the main pranayama where all the 3 bandhas are locked together while you perform retention
Utkata	intense, fierce
Utthita	extended

V

Vajra	diamond or thunderbolt
Vamadeva	a sage
Vasana	cluster of desires
Vayu	one of the vital air "wind"
Vedanta	one of the 6 orthodox schools of Hindu Philosophy, it is based on the doctrine of Upanishads
Viloma	against the current stream "against the hair"
Virabhadra	warrior
Vishuddhi	situated behind the throat

Y

Yantra	geometrical symbol for visualization

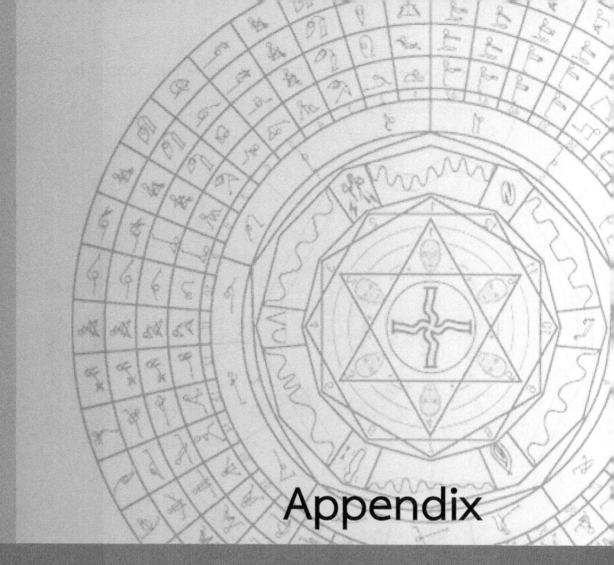

Appendix

4 x 4 Universal Yoga® Mandala Sequence

4 x 4 Universal Yoga® Mandala Sequence created by Andrey Lappa

(Start of Warm-up Set)

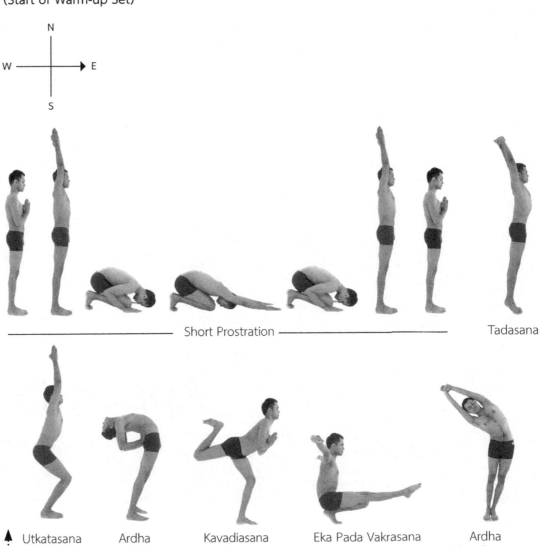

Short Prostration — Tadasana

Utkatasana   Ardha   Kavadiasana   Eka Pada Vakrasana   Ardha
            Chakrasana   Chandrasana

Mirror Reflect- Change Sides

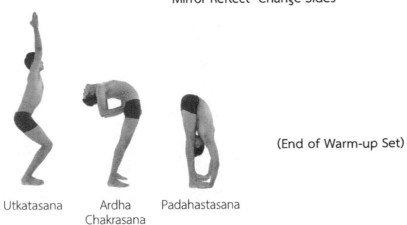

Utkatasana   Ardha   Padahastasana
            Chakrasana

(End of Warm-up Set)

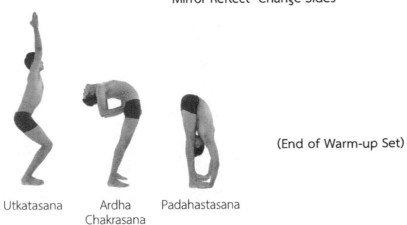

280

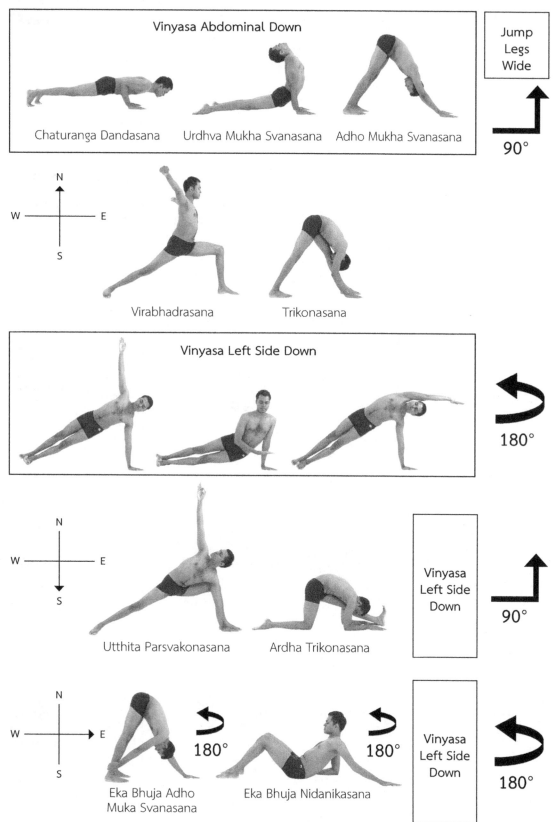

Vinyasa Abdominal Down

Chaturanga Dandasana   Urdhva Mukha Svanasana   Adho Mukha Svanasana

Jump Legs Wide

90°

N
W ——— E
S

Virabhadrasana   Trikonasana

Vinyasa Left Side Down

180°

N
W ——— E
S

Utthita Parsvakonasana   Ardha Trikonasana

Vinyasa Left Side Down

90°

N
W ——→ E
S

Eka Bhuja Adho Muka Svanasana   180°   Eka Bhuja Nidanikasana   180°

Vinyasa Left Side Down

180°

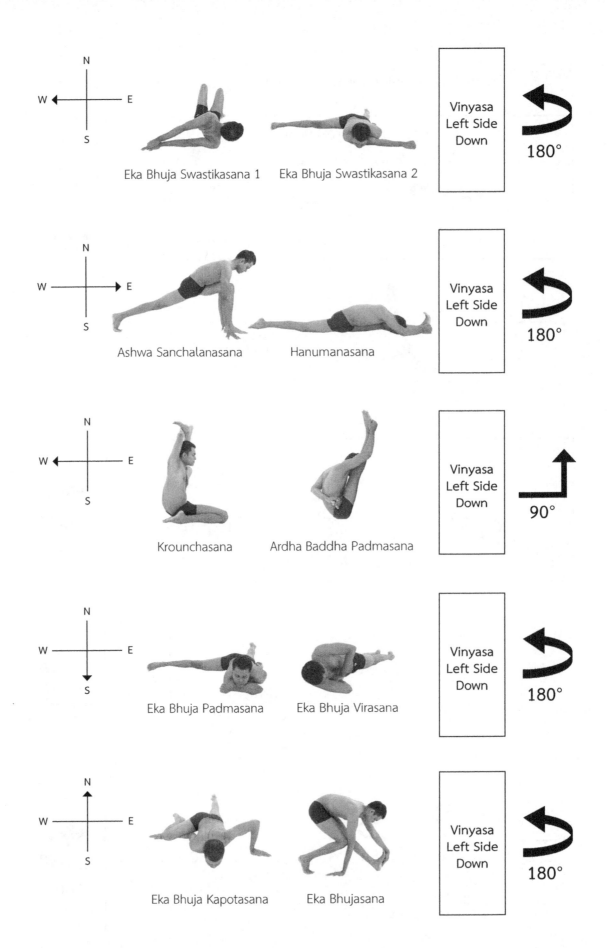

Eka Bhuja Swastikasana 1   Eka Bhuja Swastikasana 2   Vinyasa Left Side Down   180°

Ashwa Sanchalanasana   Hanumanasana   Vinyasa Left Side Down   180°

Krounchasana   Ardha Baddha Padmasana   Vinyasa Left Side Down   90°

Eka Bhuja Padmasana   Eka Bhuja Virasana   Vinyasa Left Side Down   180°

Eka Bhuja Kapotasana   Eka Bhujasana   Vinyasa Left Side Down   180°

282

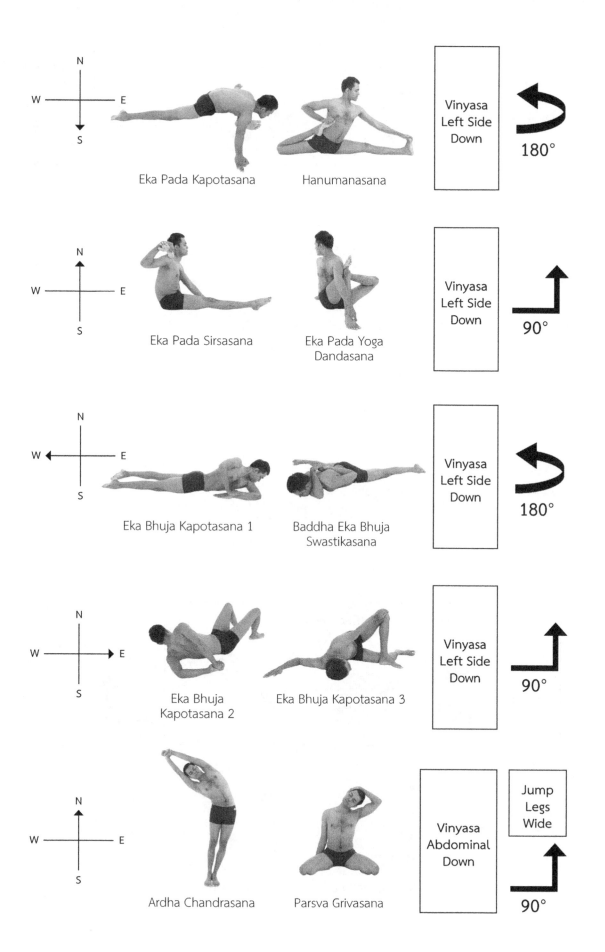

Eka Pada Kapotasana	Hanumanasana	Vinyasa Left Side Down	180°
Eka Pada Sirsasana	Eka Pada Yoga Dandasana	Vinyasa Left Side Down	90°
Eka Bhuja Kapotasana 1	Baddha Eka Bhuja Swastikasana	Vinyasa Left Side Down	180°
Eka Bhuja Kapotasana 2	Eka Bhuja Kapotasana 3	Vinyasa Left Side Down	90°
Ardha Chandrasana	Parsva Grivasana	Vinyasa Abdominal Down	Jump Legs Wide / 90°

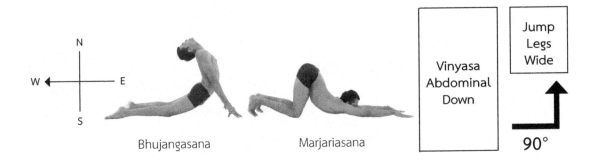

N · W · E · S

Bhujangasana   Marjariasana

Vinyasa
Abdominal
Down

Jump
Legs
Wide

90°

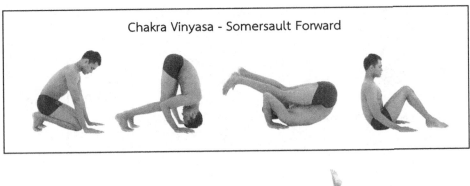

Chakra Vinyasa - Somersault Forward

N · W · E · S

Parivrtta Janu Sirsasana   Ardha Nirlamba
                                   Sarvangasana

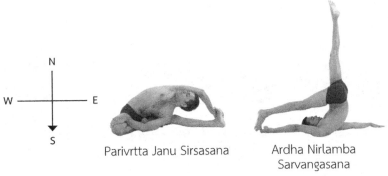

Ardha Chakra Vinyasa - Half Somersault Backward

Jump
Legs
Wide

90°

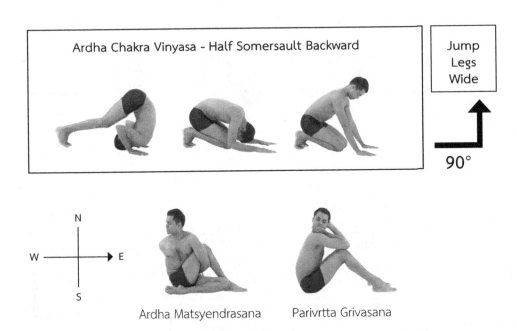

N · W · E · S

Ardha Matsyendrasana   Parivrtta Grivasana

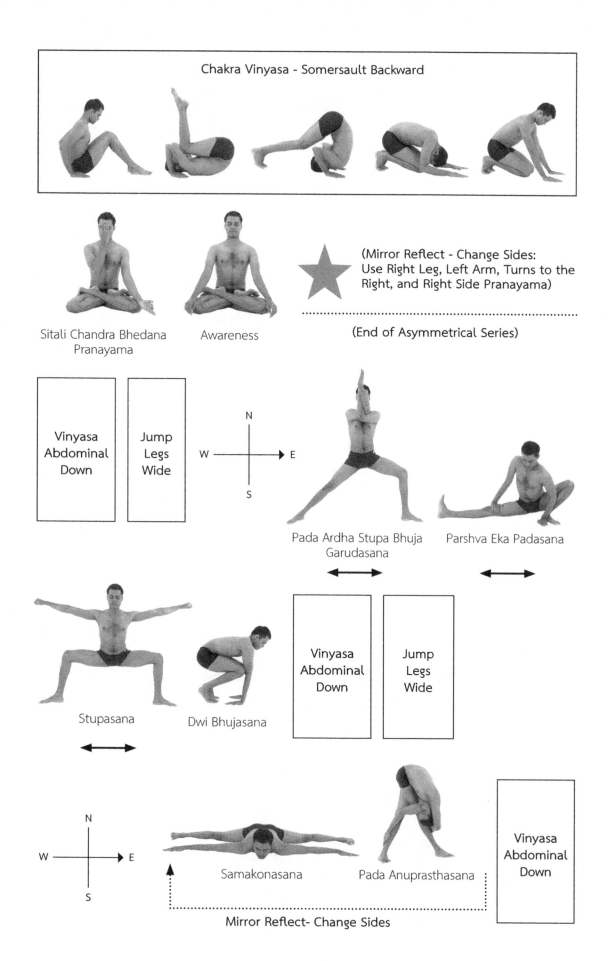

Chakra Vinyasa - Somersault Backward

Sitali Chandra Bhedana Pranayama

Awareness

(Mirror Reflect - Change Sides: Use Right Leg, Left Arm, Turns to the Right, and Right Side Pranayama)

(End of Asymmetrical Series)

Vinyasa Abdominal Down

Jump Legs Wide

N
W — E
S

Pada Ardha Stupa Bhuja Garudasana

Parshva Eka Padasana

Stupasana

Dwi Bhujasana

Vinyasa Abdominal Down

Jump Legs Wide

N
W — E
S

Samakonasana

Pada Anuprasthasana

Vinyasa Abdominal Down

Mirror Reflect- Change Sides

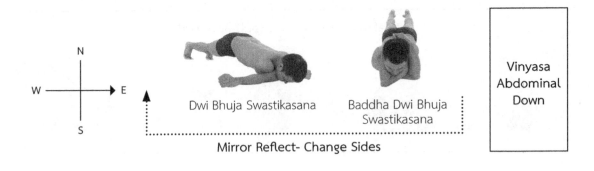

Dwi Bhuja Swastikasana

Baddha Dwi Bhuja Swastikasana

Mirror Reflect- Change Sides

Vinyasa Abdominal Down

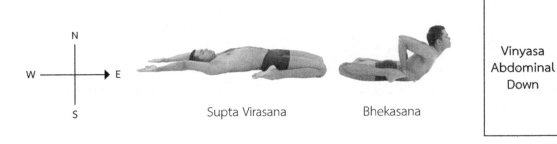

Supta Virasana

Bhekasana

Vinyasa Abdominal Down

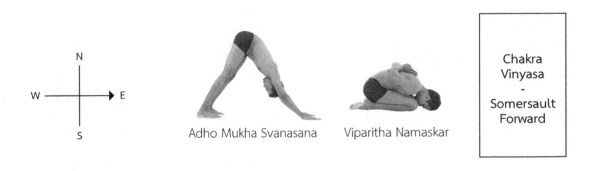

Adho Mukha Svanasana

Viparitha Namaskar

Chakra Vinyasa - Somersault Forward

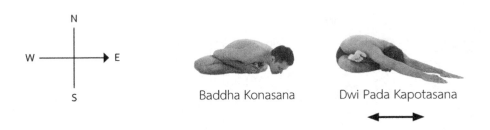

Baddha Konasana

Dwi Pada Kapotasana

Vinyasa Abdominal Up (4x)

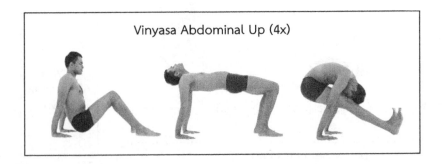

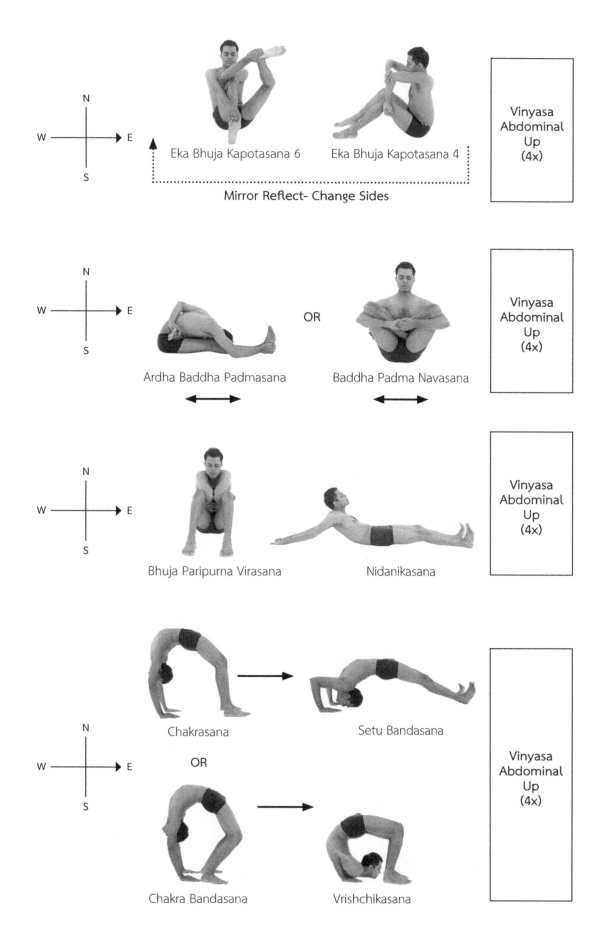

N
W → E
S

Eka Bhuja Kapotasana 6   Eka Bhuja Kapotasana 4

Mirror Reflect- Change Sides

Vinyasa
Abdominal
Up
(4x)

N
W → E
S

Ardha Baddha Padmasana   OR   Baddha Padma Navasana
↔   ↔

Vinyasa
Abdominal
Up
(4x)

N
W → E
S

Bhuja Paripurna Virasana   Nidanikasana

Vinyasa
Abdominal
Up
(4x)

Chakrasana   →   Setu Bandasana

N
W → E
S   OR

Chakra Bandasana   →   Vrishchikasana

Vinyasa
Abdominal
Up
(4x)

287

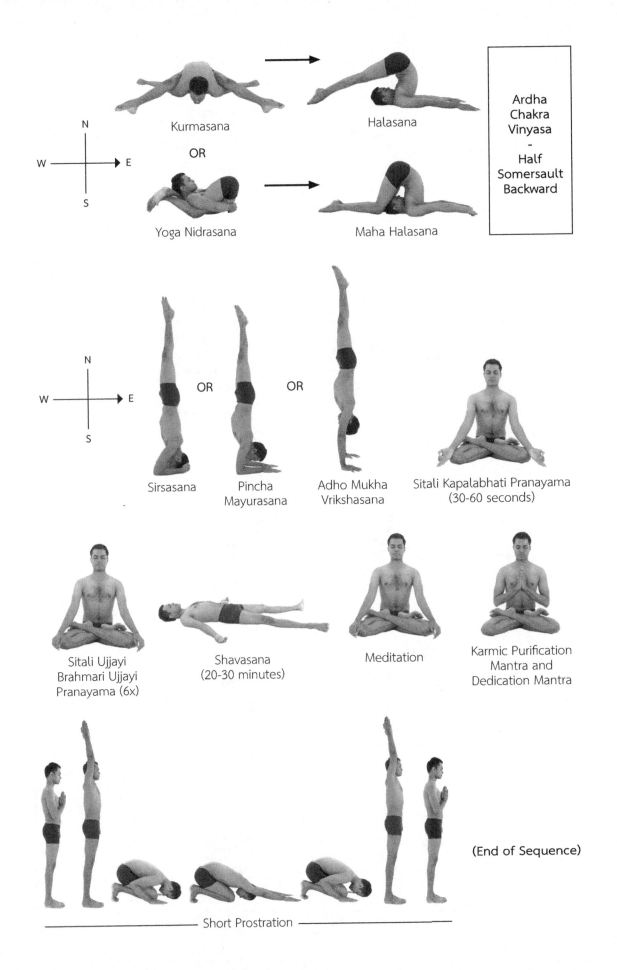

Kurmasana → Halasana

OR

Yoga Nidrasana → Maha Halasana

Ardha
Chakra
Vinyasa
-
Half
Somersault
Backward

Sirsasana OR Pincha Mayurasana OR Adho Mukha Vrikshasana

Sitali Kapalabhati Pranayama (30-60 seconds)

Sitali Ujjayi Brahmari Ujjayi Pranayama (6x)

Shavasana (20-30 minutes)

Meditation

Karmic Purification Mantra and Dedication Mantra

Short Prostration

(End of Sequence)

About the Authors

Suresh Munisamy

Suresh Munisamy is currently living in Bangkok, Thailand, where he runs his yoga center, Yoga 101, with his Thai family (www.yoga101.com). Since his childhood he has entered many competitions and won several championships and awards such as Yoga Bhooshan, Swami Vivekananda, and Yoga Vibhushan. His knowledge and discipline have helped him become one of the most highly qualified yoga educators in Asia. He has travelled widely to teach workshops and trainings on the basics of universal yoga, where he presents yoga as a tool for health and spiritual growth. He tirelessly works to focus on the change from individual transformation to collective transformation. For more information visit: www.yoga101academy.com.

Andrey Lappa

Andrey Lappa is one of the most influential yoga masters to have emerged from the post-Soviet era. Originally from Ukraine, Andrey has been practicing yoga for well over 30 years, and teaching professionally since 1988. He has studied with many well-known yoga teachers throughout the East including BKS Iyengar and Sri K. Pattabhi Jois, but also with many teachers who prefer to remain out of secular life. It is from his vast experience of travels and yoga studies that have spanned India, Nepal, Tibet, Mongolia and other Eastern Republics that Andrey developed the system called Universal Yoga®. Andrey is a recognized Lama (teacher) in the Karma Kagyu lineage, the president of the Kiev Yoga Federation, the author of Yoga: Tradition of Unification, and the author of many posters, videos, and software programs designed to transmit the yogic concepts of control, balance, creativity, karmic freedom, and ultimate liberation for all practitioners. For more information visit: www.universal-yoga.com

Made in the USA
Monee, IL
05 February 2022

89867142R00162